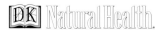

DK Natural Health.

Secrets of

BACH FLOWER REMEDIES

D1413659

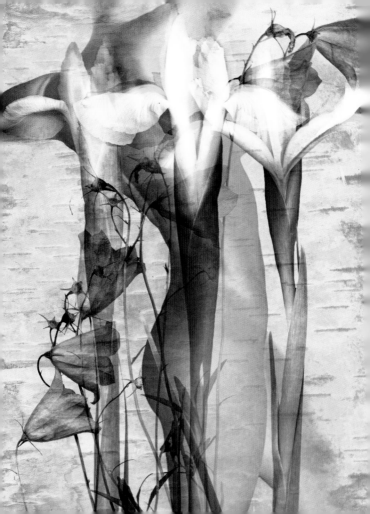

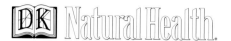

DK Natural Health.

Secrets of

BACH FLOWER REMEDIES

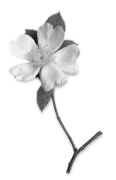

JEREMY HARWOOD

A Dorling Kindersley Book

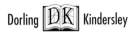

Dorling DK Kindersley

LONDON, NEW YORK, SYDNEY, DELHI, PARIS,
MUNICH and JOHANNESBURG

This book was conceived, designed, and produced by
THE IVY PRESS LIMITED,
The Old Candlemakers, Lewes, East Sussex BN7 2NZ, UK

Art director *Peter Bridgewater*
Editorial director *Sophie Collins*
Designers *Kevin Knight, Jane Lanaway*
Editor *Rowan Davies*
Picture researchers *Liz Eddison, Vanessa Fletcher*
Photography *Guy Ryecart*
Illustrations *Sarah Young, Catherine McIntyre, Vanessa Luff, Andrew Milne*
Models *Mark Jamieson*

First published in The United States of America in 2000 by
DORLING KINDERSLEY PUBLISHING, INC.,
95 Madison Avenue, New York, New York 10016

Natural Health ® is a registered trademark of Weider
Publications, Inc. *Natural Health* magazine is the
leading publication in the field of natural self-care. For
subscription information call 800–526–8440 or visit
www.naturalhealthmag.com

Library of Congress Cataloging-in-Publication Data

Harwood, Jeremy
The secrets of Bach flower remedies/Jeremy Harwood.
    p. cm.
Includes index.
ISBN 0-7894-6774-7 (alk. paper)
1. Flowers--Therapeutic use. I. Title.
RX615.F55 H36 2000
615'.321--dc21

                                              00-057063

Originated and printed by
Hong Kong Graphic and Printing Limited, China

see our complete
catalog at
www.dk.com

CONTENTS

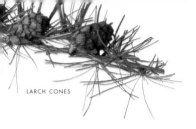

LARCH CONES

HOW TO USE THIS BOOK To make

Secrets of Bach Flower Remedies easy to use, it has been deliberately split into two distinct sections. The first of these provides you with the essential background, so that you can understand what the Bach system of healing is, how it works, and how the remedies it consists of are prepared and taken. The second—the core of the book—is an remedy-by-remedy guide, subdivided into the emotional groups that Dr. Bach devised for his final book, *The Twelve Healers and Other Remedies*.

Important Notice

If you suffer from anxiety, depression, or any emotional problems that are seriously affecting your work, social life or relationships you should seek the advice of your registered medical practitioner. It is also important to inform your doctor of any remedies or medications you are taking. If you ever feel that you might do harm to yourself or others you must seek immediate medical attention. You must also seek urgent medical attention if you experience unusual or unexplained symptoms, particularly involving a loss of consciousness.

Do not use Bach Flower Remedies to replace medical treatment you are receiving for severe problems.

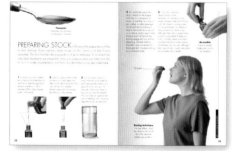

Practical information
Practical pages like these tell you how the remedies are prepared and how best to take them.

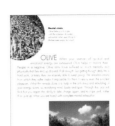

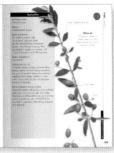

OLIVE

Plant guides

Coverage of each remedy starts with a guide to the plant from which it comes.

Detail

More detailed pages supplement the guides, telling you more about the remedy, how it works, and the emotional states it can treat.

Key

Icons show you to which group each remedy belongs.

FEAR

UNCERTAINTY

LACK OF INTEREST

LONELINESS

OVER-SENSITIVITY

DESPAIR

OVER-ANXIETY

The Aspen Remedy

Courage

A severe state

REMEDIES IN ACTION

Case Study

Case Study

Case Study

Application

Other features include question and answer pages and case studies to show the remedies in action.

Introduction

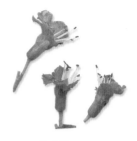

Red Chestnut
Red Chestnut flowers are just one of the 38 flower remedies Dr. Bach discovered and researched.

Dr. Edward Bach (1886–1936), the discoverer of the celebrated flower remedies, was a Harley Street, London, doctor who abandoned orthodox medicine to become a pioneer medical revolutionary.

Dissatisfied with the conventional approach to the diagnosis and treatment of disease he had learned at medical school and later put into use during his years as a hospital doctor and in his Harley Street practice, Dr. Bach turned firstly to homeopathy. He believed, with Samuel Hahnemann, the founding father of the therapy, that "the patient is the most important factor in his healing." He won a considerable reputation in this field—the vaccines, known as Bach nosodes, that he isolated still play a valuable role in homeopathy today—but this was not enough to satisfy him and his high ideals.

A unique system of healing

Homeopathy and personal experience had taught Dr. Bach much, but he wanted more. Eventually, he decided to strike out to develop what was to become a unique system of healing of his own. He began work on this in the 1920s and continued with it almost up to his death in 1936, which took place shortly after he had completed the final revision of his seminal work, *The Twelve Healers and Other Remedies*. This is an essential starting point for anyone who wants to find out more about the Bach system of healing and how it works. It is clear, and eminently straightforward. This is not surprising when you realize that one of Bach's main ideals throughout his working life was the need to make things simple. The remedies he discovered, as he himself put it, were derived from "simple" herbs, and the system of healing, of which they formed the basis, was equally simple.

Dr. Bach was determined that, as he said, "without a knowledge of medicine" the remedies and how to employ them could "be understood so easily that they can be used in any household." In the same 1936 lecture, which he delivered on his 50th birthday, he went on to stress that: "It is not the disease that is of importance, *it is the patient*, the way in which he or she is affected, which is our true guide to healing."

Followers of the Bach system believe it to be complete in itself, and find that it benefits their health. However, do not use the remedies to replace any regular medication, and if you see no improvement in your condition after two to three weeks, stop taking the remedy. Consult your doctor before you embark on a course of remedies, or if you suffer any unfamiliar symptoms.

EDWARD BACH
THE MAN AND HIS FLOWERS

Dr. Edward Bach—the name, by the way, is pronounced "Batch"—must have been a fascinating man to know. The amazing thing, in fact, is that we know so much about his work, for he left relatively little in the form of permanent research records behind. This was an act of deliberate omission. Once Dr. Bach had completed his final work on his system of healing, he burned most of his notes as part of his policy of keeping things as simple as possible. The system, as it now stood, was perfect—and there was no point at all in complicating matters by introducing the possibility of confusion. In this opening section of *Secrets of Bach Flower Remedies*, you will find out more about the man and his philosophy, how the remedies he discovered are prepared, and how people are treated—or treat themselves—with them.

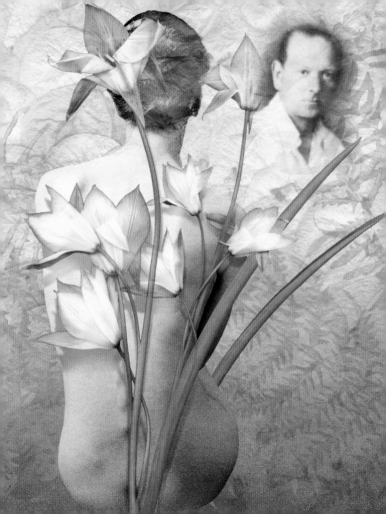

The Bach Remedies

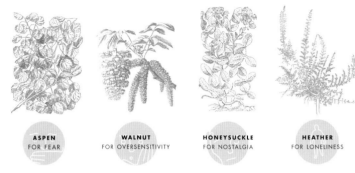

ASPEN
FOR FEAR

WALNUT
FOR OVERSENSITIVITY

HONEYSUCKLE
FOR NOSTALGIA

HEATHER
FOR LONELINESS

The 38 flower remedies—39 with the addition of Rescue Remedy—that Dr. Edward Bach discovered make up a unique system of healing that is complete in itself. With thorough and painstaking research, he devised his flower remedies to be effective against every possible negative state of mind—taken singly or in combination, they had the ability to help people to counteract such problems, with the result that any unwelcome physical conditions would be helped as well. Bach believed firmly that physical ill-health was a result of an imbalance within the mind. Whatever the problem, therefore, the driving forces behind the selection of specific remedies were the emotional outlook, mood, temperament, and personality of the individual concerned. "Treat the patient according to the mood, according to the character, and individuality and you cannot go wrong." He also added that disease in itself was of no consequence whatsoever since it was "the manner in which a patient reacts to an illness that alone should be taken into account."

The other Bach watchword was simplicity, his stated aim being to devise a method of choosing which remedies to give that was "simple enough for most people to understand." It was this

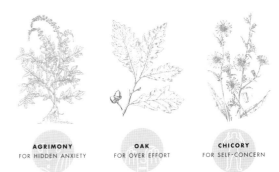

AGRIMONY
FOR HIDDEN ANXIETY

OAK
FOR OVER EFFORT

CHICORY
FOR SELF-CONCERN

passion for simplicity that led him to review and refine his approach, until he was ready with the final version of the great system of healing.

Refining the system
Studying Dr. Bach's few surviving writings gives an indication of what he was doing: you will notice, for example, how he eventually abandoned the schemes he had initially devised to classify the remedies he had discovered over the years. Now, he split all 38 remedies into seven groups, which he categorized as being for: fear, uncertainty, insufficient interest in present circumstances, loneliness, oversensitivity to influences and ideas, despondency or despair, and being overanxious for the welfare of others. By studying the groups, you will have all the information you need to use the Bach system.

The one further division that remains is between what Dr. Bach termed mood and type remedies. Basically, all 38 remedies can be taken to improve mood, but some, in addition, are type remedies—that is to say, they are specifically suited to helping different personality types.

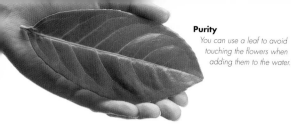

Purity

You can use a leaf to avoid touching the flowers when adding them to the water.

THE SUN METHOD

To create what he termed "mother tinctures," Dr. Bach devised two preparation methods: the first relies on the action of the sun; the second on boiling twigs, leaves and flowers in pure springwater (see pages 18–19). The sun method, which is unique to flower therapy, is used for flowers that come into bloom during the late spring and summer, when the sun is at the height of its power. You will need a plain glass or crystal bowl, a small glass jug, a dropper bottle, scissors, and brandy. You may also need a bigger bottle for bottled still mineral water or springwater if there is no clear, unpolluted running water near where the flowers are growing. The jug, scissors, bowl, and bottles should be sterilized in advance.

Equipment

The glassware that is needed for remedy preparation is simple and straightforward to obtain.

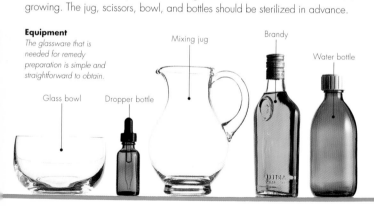

Glass bowl   Dropper bottle   Mixing jug   Brandy   Water bottle

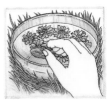

1 The flowers should be picked at around 9 AM, when their blooms are freshly opened and at their best. Fill a bowl with pure springwater and remove the flowerheads so that they fall directly into it. The aim is to float blossoms on the surface of the water until it is thickly covered—the blooms may overlap as long as they all touch the water. Avoid touching the water or the flowers yourself or casting a shadow over the bowl. Leave it to stand in full sunshine for three hours—or until the blooms show signs of fading. During this time the water is becoming energized.

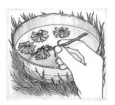

2 Discard the flower-heads, taking care not to touch the surface of the water as you do so.

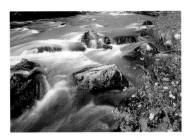

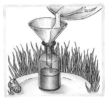

3 The final step involves mixing, in the dropper bottle, the energized water 50:50 with 40 percent proof brandy to make the mother tincture. Brandy was Dr. Bach's own choice of preservative and is the one that the Bach Centre still uses today. If you are concerned about using alcohol, it is worth noting that the remedy you take is so diluted that the amount of alcohol in it is infinitesimal. The mother tincture retains its strength indefinitely.

Permission
You may need landowner's permission to pick wild flowers. Never pick flowers you cannot identify—they may be rare and protected.

Energizing
The mixture needs to stand for several hours for the water to be energized.

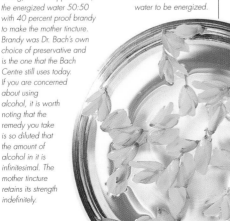

The Man Who Discovered Flower Remedies

Had Dr. Edward Bach stuck to his Harley Street office in London, his name would probably feature as an extended footnote in the story of complementary medicine, largely thanks to his discovery of the seven Bach nosodes, homeopathic vaccines that are still used in modern homeopathy. However, Bach's enquiring mind led him to strike out on a new path that was totally his own, earning him a unique position in the story of natural healing.

Underlying Bach's beliefs was his notion that illness and disease were not primarily the result of physical causes. Rather, they were due to a deeper internal disharmony resulting from emotional imbalance.

What Bach believed

Bach came to believe that emotional factors, such as fear and anxiety, led to distress of mind and that this depleted the body's natural vitality, with a consequent loss of natural resistance. He concluded that, instead of simply treating physical symptoms, it was essential to eliminate the cause of the problem which, in most cases, was either mental or spiritual. His ultimate ambition was to devise a truly

1886	1912	1917	1919
Bach born in Moseley, Warwickshire.	Completes medical studies, qualifies, and starts to practice.	Given only a few months to live by his medical colleagues following operation for cancer.	Appointed to the London Homeopathic Hospital.

CERATO

BACH AS A YOUNG MAN

CHERRY PLUM

comprehensive system of treatment that would deal with disease by resolving emotional imbalances directly.

Discovering how to divide people into personality groups, according to character and behavior, was one key development. The other was the discovery of a trigger that would act to alter existing mental or spiritual states positively. In this context Bach was looking for a purer form of medicine that would be wholly positive in its actions, and for this he turned to wild plants and flowers. In 1928 he discovered the first two flower remedies and, in 1930, abandoned his London practice to devote himself to searching for more remedies and perfecting his new system of healing.

Over the next four years, Bach discovered 17 more remedies. Having settled in Mount Vernon, in Sotwell, southern England, he set to work again, looking for further remedies. By August 1935, he had identified another 19. As Bach had intended, the flower remedies that he had discovered and the simple methods of working with them that he had developed were soon on the way to placing the ability to heal in the hands of all.

1928	1934	1936
Discovers the first two flower remedies in Wales. Two years later, leaves his London office for good.	Sets up permanent home at Mount Vernon, Oxfordshire, where he continues his research.	Dies in November, having completed his final work on the flower remedies.

DR. BACH

CHICORY

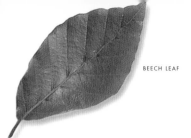

BEECH LEAF

THE BOILING METHOD

Dr. Bach's sun preparation method (see pages 14–15) is still used today to prepare 20 of the Bach flower remedies. For the other 18, most of which are made with tougher flowering twigs, Bach devised the boiling method. For this you will need a stainless-steel or enamel pot with a lid, pruning-shears, two small glass jugs, a dropper bottle, still mineral or springwater, brandy, and two or three pieces of filter paper. The pot, jugs, shears, and dropper bottle must be all sterilized.

Equipment

The equipment needs to be sterilized before use by boiling the various items gently in clean water in the pot. You should allow around 20 minutes for this.

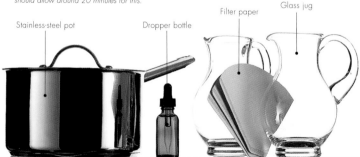

Stainless-steel pot

Dropper bottle

Filter paper

Glass jug

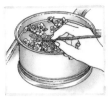 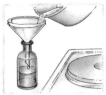

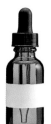

1 Gather the flowering sprays, leaves and twigs early on a sunny morning. Drop them into a pot without touching them. When the pot is about three-quarters full put the lid on. Once at home, cover the flowers and twigs with still mineral or springwater—and boil them—uncovered—for half an hour. Put the lid on and let the saucepan stand in the fresh air until the energized water is cold, before removing the twigs, leaves and flowers. Let it stand a little longer to give any sediment a chance to settle.

2 Finally, cover one of the jugs with filter paper. Fill the other jug with the energized water and pour it, a little at a time, onto to the filter paper, repeating the process until enough water has been filtered to half-fill the dropper bottle, which you have already half-filled with brandy. Add the water to the brandy to make the mother tincture.

Labelling
Label the tincture bottle carefully including name, date, and place.

Standing time
Allow the energized water to stand to let sediment settle.

Heating
You could use a portable gas burner to heat the pot on site.

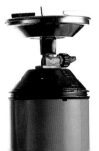

Sediment

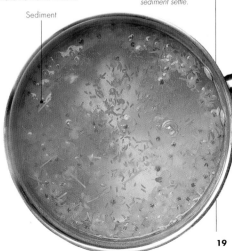

Which Flowers, Which Method?

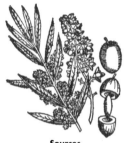

Sources
Olive is one of three Bach flower remedies that originate outside Britain, the others being Vine and Cerato.

With the exceptions of Olive, Vine, and Cerato, all the plants that are used to prepare the flower remedies grow in the wild on sites scattered throughout England and Wales, just as they did when Dr. Bach first set about investigating their healing powers in 1928. Of the 38 basic remedies, all but one come from flowers or plants, the exception being Rock Water, which is a specially prepared natural springwater.

Bach devised two natural ways of harnessing the healing potency of the flowers to create the mother tinctures—the sun method (see pages 14–15) and the boiling method (see pages 18–19).

The drawback of the sun method is that it can be used only for flowers that bloom during late spring and summer, when the sun is at its strongest. He quickly found that in the early spring in the northern hemisphere the sun was not strong enough for the sun method to be employed to energize the water successfully. So he devised the boiling method, which involves boiling flowers, catkins, and twigs of trees, bushes and plants, most of which bloom early in the year before there is much sunshine.

The chart shows which flowers are prepared by which method, together with when to prepare them. The exact times vary, depending on the weather. Olive and Vine flowering times vary depending on the flowering season in the countries in which they grow.

Preparation		
Cherry Plum	late winter to mid-spring	BOILING
Elm	early to mid-spring	BOILING
Aspen	early to mid-spring	BOILING
Beech	mid- to late spring	BOILING
Chestnut Bud	mid- to late spring	BOILING
Hornbeam	mid- to late spring	BOILING
Larch	mid- to late spring	BOILING
Walnut	mid- to late spring	BOILING
Oak	mid- to late spring	SUN
Star of Bethlehem	mid-spring to early summer	BOILING
Gorse	mid-spring to early summer	SUN
Holly	late spring	BOILING
Crab Apple	late spring	BOILING
Willow	late spring	BOILING
Olive	late spring	SUN
Vine	late spring	SUN
Red Chestnut	late spring to early summer	BOILING
Pine	late spring to early summer	BOILING
White Chestnut	late spring to early summer	SUN
Water Violet	late spring to early summer	SUN
Mustard	late spring to midsummer	BOILING
Rock Water	early to midsummer	SUN
Honeysuckle	early to late summer	BOILING
Sweet Chestnut	early to late summer	BOILING
Wild Rose	early to late summer	BOILING
Mimulus	early to late summer	SUN
Agrimony	early to late summer	SUN
Scleranthus	early to late summer	SUN
Rock Rose	early summer to early fall	SUN
Centaury	early summer to early fall	SUN
Wild Oat	mid- to late summer	SUN
Impatiens	midsummer to early fall	SUN
Chicory	midsummer to early fall	SUN
Vervain	midsummer to early fall	SUN
Clematis	midsummer to early fall	SUN
Heather	midsummer to early fall	SUN
Cerato	late summer to early fall	SUN
Gentian	late summer to early fall	SUN

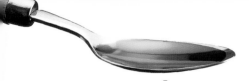

Teaspoon
Remedies can be taken in a teaspoon of water.

USING THE FLOWER REMEDIES

Following the preparation of the mother tincture, there are two more stages in the creation of the flower remedies. The first involves the preparation of stock remedies, from which the individual treatments are prepared. How you prepare what you take from the stock is a matter of preference and there are alternative ways described here.

1 *To make up a stock bottle—this is the sort of bottle that you will find on sale through Bach remedy distributors—fill a sterilized 1oz (30ml) dropper bottle with brandy.*

2 *Add two drops of the mother tincture to it. It may seem very little, but Dr. Bach found that this was all that was needed. Adding more will not improve the efficacy of the remedy.*

3 *You can simply add two drops from the stock bottle of each appropriate remedy to a glass of water and sip it at intervals at least four times a day until you feel the benefits. This would be an appropriate way of dealing with a passing negative mood, for example.*

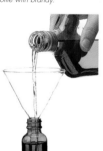

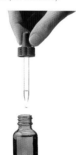

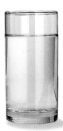

4 You could also place the drops straight on the tongue, take them in a teaspoon of water, or add them to a cup of tea, coffee, or other beverage. You should aim to hold each dose in the mouth for a second or so before swallowing it while thinking about all the positive healing energy that you will be absorbing. Another method, probably more convenient for the longer term, involves making up a treatment bottle.

5 To do this, place two drops of each of the remedies you are taking in an empty dropper bottle and fill it up with still mineral water or spring-water. It is recommended you take four drops at least four times a day, although there are no upper limits, since it is impossible to take too much. Similarly, there is no hard and fast restriction on the number of remedies you can use, although Bach practitioners usually advocate no more than six or seven.

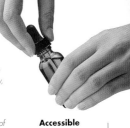

Accessible
Carry an remedy bottle with you for convenience.

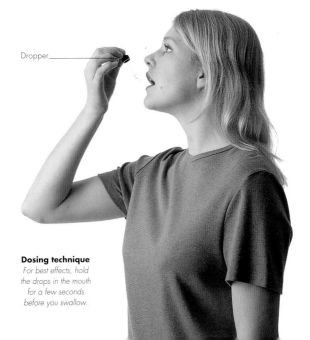

Dropper

Dosing technique
For best effects, hold the drops in the mouth for a few seconds before you swallow.

Healing Fundamentals

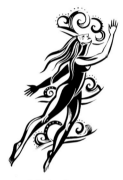

Self-development
The remedies help to encourage the development of the "higher self."

Making the flower remedies is a simple process that does not demand any special abilities. Deciding on which flower remedies to take for what, how much of them to take, and for how long, should be a straightforward process. One of Dr. Bach's aims was to avoid anything that seemed overcomplex. As he wrote to his friend and colleague Victor Bullen shortly before his death,

"Our work is steadfastly to adhere to the simplicity and purity of this method of healing." At about the same time, Bach burned many of his research notes. In his mind, the discarded research, like the theories he had abandoned as his work progressed, had now outlived their purpose. All that it was necessary to say, he believed, was now set down in the final version of his work: *The Twelve Healers and Other Remedies.*

In matters of health and healing, the key, Bach held, comes from self-knowledge. This involves building an understanding of what he termed the "higher self"—the spiritual side—and the everyday personality. If the spiritual side and the personality diverge, the result is an imbalance, with layer after layer of negative emotion building up.

This is what Bach practitioners term the snowball effect. It can occur if, for instance, we are living counter to our inner natures, or if we choose to take a course of action that upsets others—and ultimately ourselves. The resulting inner

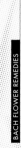

imbalance and emotional turmoil can lead to ill-health. Deal with the imbalance and tackle the emotional difficulties and the physical problems are also on the way to being resolved.

Stripping away the layers

The aim of treatment is to strip away these layers of negative emotion until the core problem is uncovered, so that it, too, can be resolved. This is exactly what taking the appropriate Bach remedies achieves. Their restorative powers act to resolve the situation in a process Bach practitioners term "peeling the onion." As layer after layer is peeled away, the problems can be tackled one by one as they are exposed. It is a process of self-exploration that psychologists will tell you can be extremely valuable.

As Dr. Bach put it, the remedies are like "beautiful music," their action serving to "open up our channels for reception of our spiritual self," so encouraging and strengthening the positive emotions we all possess.

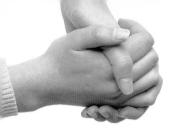

Signs of stress
Clasping the hands together and wringing them can be a sign of inner stress.

CONSULTING

With the Bach system of healing it is more than just acceptable to diagnose and treat yourself—it is a step that qualified Bach practitioners actively encourage you to take. It involves getting to know what each of the remedies is for, which occasionally can be a little more complicated than it might initially appear. Sometimes, however, if problems seem so complex that you cannot see your way through them, seeking help and advice from a practitioner is the obvious step to take.

Diagnosis

For a Bach practitioner, a knowledge and understanding of basic body language and what it may signify can be extremely helpful in making a diagnosis. Sometimes, it can reveal the presence of inner tensions of which the patient may be unaware, or ones which he or she finds it hard to quantify and explain verbally. In such a case, your body can be your best friend.

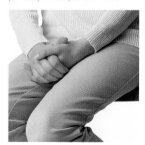

Practitioner

To find a competent practitioner, start by consulting the useful addresses (see page 221). The Dr. Edward Bach Foundation registers trained practitioners who agree to work to a strict code of conduct. You will also find the names and addresses of Bach remedy distributors throughout the world. Alternatively, enquire at a local health food store or pharmacy.

Consultation

Before you agree to a consultation, find out how much it will cost, how long it will take, and exactly what it will include. Normally, an initial consultation takes around an hour and the charge includes mixing up a suitable treatment bottle. You also should check how the remedies will be selected and whether or not the practitioner uses genuine ones.

Trust

Establishing a trusting relationship between patient and practitioner is important.

Mental state

What is going on in your mind is more important than physical symptoms.

Listening is more important than talking

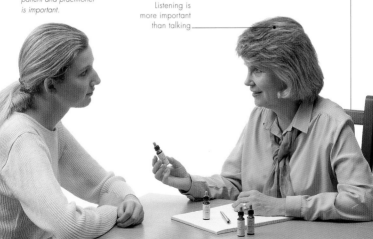

27

Making a Diagnosis

Listening and talking are the two keys to determining which remedies it is appropriate to suggest. The process should be a straightforward one, reflecting the simplicity of the Bach system of healing. As a starting point, the practitioner may ask you what you know about the flower remedies. This may lead to a short explanation of the system itself. The next step is to find out why you are there and to identify what your problems are. You should stress how you feel at that moment, since treatment starts by stripping away what is currently troubling you before identifying and treating other deeper negative emotions, if they are present.

First and foremost, the practitioner's job is to listen to what you are saying. In the main, questions should be used to help to clarify and amplify what you are discussing, though, at times, the practitioner may try to steer the conversation in a particular direction. This could be to open up an area that might be important to diagnosis and

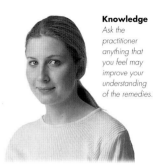

Knowledge
Ask the practitioner anything that you feel may improve your understanding of the remedies.

treatment, or the aim could be to help you to clarify your thoughts and then discuss what you are feeling openly and frankly.

Question and answer

Some practitioners might probe into what depression or stress mean to you, while others might ask you how you would act in a given situation. Such questions help practitioners understand what kind of person you are, pointing them toward the type remedy that is considered appropriate. Near the end of the consultation, the practitioner will sum up what he or she has understood.

After giving you the chance to comment, he or she will suggest appropriate remedies. Here, the most important thing is for you to feel reassured by what is being selected, which involves asking about what has prompted each suggested selection. The answer should be that these remedies will help to bring all of your various positive qualities to the fore. Finally, your appropriate treatment bottle will be mixed.

This is all that a true Bach consultation should involve. Some practitioners, however, believe that other diagnostic techniques, such as psychometry, kinesiology, radiesthesia and dowsing, can also help in remedy selection. This merely cloaks the process in unnecessary mystery.

Dosage

Unless you are advised otherwise by your practitioner, the usual dosage for the remedies is four drops, taken at regular intervals throughout the day.

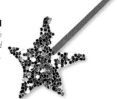

A magic wand
Rescue Remedy is the emergency "magic" wand of all the Bach remedies.

SELF-DIAGNOSIS

When you use the Bach system, you are concerned solely with emotional states and personality problems; this means setting aside any physical symptoms. Your selection of remedies should be based on how you feel currently, not on how you think you felt in the past. You should treat only what you see, rather than trying to deal with too much too soon. Before embarking on any form of self-diagnosis or self-prescribed treatment, it is always advisable to discuss your symptoms with your registered medical practitioner.

Choosing a remedy
Start by identifying your mood and then, by cross-referring to what each of the 38 remedies is intended to treat, find the matching mood remedy. List all the appropriate remedies by applying the principles given above. Rank the remaining remedies in order of importance. A single remedy may be enough, but it may be better to try a selection. In such cases, the appropriate type remedy—the one that best reflects your underlying character—is often included with the mood remedies. Looking at the way you react to specific situations will provide you with valuable clues to your character.

GOOD FAIRY

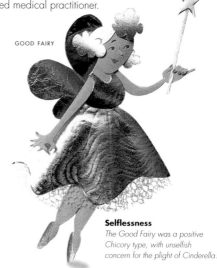

Selflessness
The Good Fairy was a positive Chicory type, with unselfish concern for the plight of Cinderella.

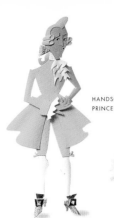

HANDSOME
PRINCE

Malice

*To counteract their
malice for Cinderella
the Ugly Stepsisters
should have taken Holly.*

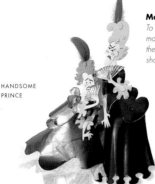

UGLY STEPSISTERS

Panic

*Rock Rose may have eased the
Prince's panic at the thought of
never finding his Princess again.*

Character types

Many teachers of Bach Flower
Remedies have suggested that tying
the main characters in well-known
fairy tales to their character type
was a useful way of getting to
know the remedies better. It is also
a way of helping you to improve
your self-diagnostic skills.
Cinderella herself was obviously
a Centaury type, put upon by
her overbearing stepsisters and
seemingly unable to resist their
demands and stand up for herself.
You need not confine yourself to
fairy tales, of course—other
practitioners suggest trying
the same thing with famous
Shakespearean plays, such
as *Hamlet*.

Enslavement

*Cinderella was a
typical Centaury type
(very put upon and
unable to stand up
for herself).*

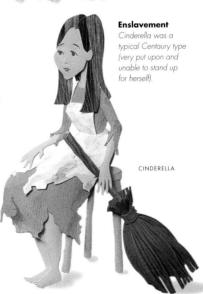

CINDERELLA

Pregnancy and Birth

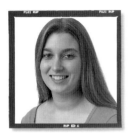

Stress in pregnancy
*Many pregnant women find that
the remedies help with stress.*

Both pregnancy and childbirth are natural, normal conditions. There are times during both when moods, feelings, and states of mind fluctuate more than usual. This is where Bach flower therapy can come into its own. The rewards are obvious—achieving a quiet, contented state of mind is one of the best ways to prepare for giving birth. Nor is the expectant mother the sole beneficiary of the Bach treatment since counteracting negative mood swings and reestablishing emotional balance and inner harmony clearly benefit the developing baby in the womb.

During pregnancy there are specific circumstances when certain remedies may be more appropriate than others. Rescue Remedy, in particular, can prove invaluable, especially as you approach and enter labor. Many women who have taken it for a few days before giving birth say that it not only makes the process far less stressful but also helps them to recover faster afterward.

Babies, too, can benefit from the action of the remedies. It is impossible to overdose on them and they have no adverse side effects. In fact, it may be easier to prescribe for babies and small children, since they tend not to conceal or suppress their emotions. There is no reason to worry about the alcohol used in the preparation of the remedies, since the actual amount involved is microscopic. A standard treatment bottle contains six teaspoons (30 milliliters) of water, plus a mere two drops of each selected remedy, and an individual dose consists of only four drops. Even a small baby will not be affected by such a small amount.

Case Study

Roberta's problems came to a head just after giving birth to her daughter, when she and her husband separated. Since then, she has been going through major ups and downs, feeling in control of her emotions one minute and totally out of control the next. Her great fear is the effect her separation will have on her baby and her other children, and their future well-being.

Red Chestnut was suggested to help Roberta cope with her constant concerns about her children's possible reactions to the situation, and the effect it was having on them.

White Chestnut was advised to ease her mental torment, and **Olive** to help deal with her physical and mental exhaustion.

Oak was advised to give her the energy she needed to carry on, together with **Elm** to stop her feeling so overwhelmed and to give her confidence, and **Star of Bethlehem** for the shock of the whole situation.

Subsequently, **Sweet Chestnut** was added to help her with her despair, **Scleranthus** to assist with decisions, and **Honeysuckle** to aid her in breaking free from the ties of the past. After just one month, the remedies were starting to take effect. Roberta had started to get her life in order, feel better about herself, and look forward to the future.

DIRECTORY
A FLOWER-BY-FLOWER GUIDE

The detailed descriptions that follow tell you everything you need to know about the individual flowers and plants that Dr. Bach identified as being the essential components of his unique system of healing. They are grouped in seven separate categories, following the masterplan laid out in his seminal work. If you decide to try making your own remedies, you should ensure that the plants you use are exactly the same botanically as the ones originally identified and prescribed by Dr. Bach. Substituting others means that the resulting remedies will not work as they should. You should also be aware that, even if the plants are botanically correct, differences in soil and climate can also limit the effectiveness of whatever you prepare.

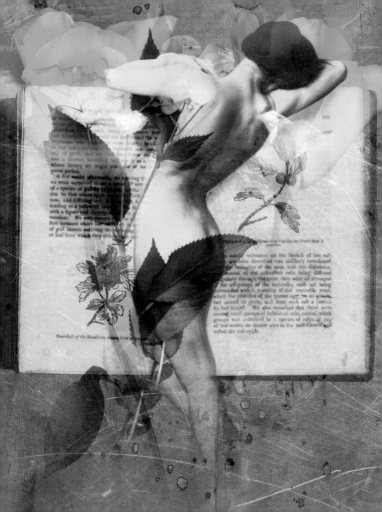

Remedies for Fear

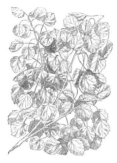

Fear of the unknown
There are many different kinds of fear. Take Aspen for unknown fears.

Fear is something everyone suffers from at various times and to varying degrees. It may be something as concrete as fear of the consequences of an injury or illness or fear of losing your job. Equally, it can be something vague and unknown, for which there is no clear explanation or reason. To help people deal with such negative emotions, Dr. Bach grouped together five different remedies, one for each type of fear he had identified. To treat everyday fears—specifically, finite fears that can be precisely identified and named—Dr. Bach prescribed Mimulus as the primary remedy. In cases of extreme terror and hopelessness, he advised taking Rock Rose, either on its own or, if circumstances warranted it, in combination with additional remedies.

An unchanged emotion

For fear of the unknown—that is, vague, insubstantial fears for which there appears to be no logical explanation or reason—Dr. Bach's advice was to take Aspen; for fear of what he termed "reason giving way," he suggested Cherry Plum. Finally, Red Chestnut was prescribed for "those who find it difficult not to be anxious for other people." Sufferers from this form of fear, Dr. Bach believed, had often "ceased to worry about themselves." Instead, they were prone to worrying about "those of whom they are fond…frequently anticipating that some unfortunate thing may happen to them."

It is worth remembering that the beauty of the Bach system of healing lies in its simplicity. It is full, final, and complete. Arguments that life has changed so substantially for all of us since Dr. Bach's time, and that more remedies are needed, completely miss the point.

To put it at its simplest, fear today is exactly the same emotion as it has always been. Only its causes may differ. In the mid-1930s, when Dr. Bach was writing, it might have been a fear of possible war and its subsequent upheaval: equally, today, it might be fear of global environmental pollution, or of genetically modified food. The remedies remain timeless and always relevant to whatever situations we are facing.

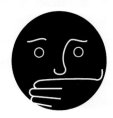

Fear

The fears you may suffer from in a negative Mimulus state are seemingly endless.

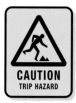

MIMULUS

Generally speaking, the remedy derived from Mimulus will help to dispel everyday fears and anxieties that can be positively identified. Examples include fear of speaking in public, fear of animals, or simply fear of the dark. People with marked negative Mimulus traits tend to be shy and nervous: frequently, they will take refuge in their own company rather than get involved in social situations. The remedy, however, will stimulate the inner reserves of strength and courage that lie concealed under surface worries and anxieties, so enabling all those common doubts and fears to be faced, learned from, and overcome.

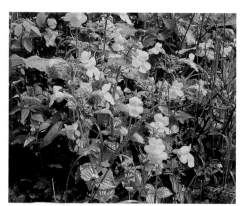

Appearance
Mimulus in full blossom. It is sometimes called the Monkey Flower.

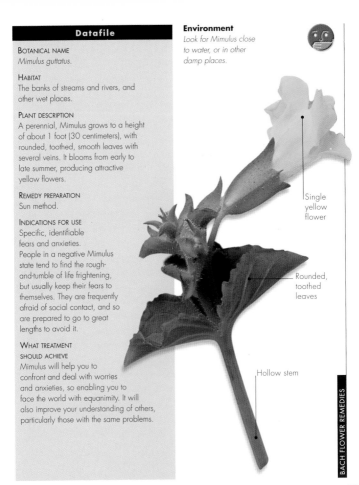

Datafile

BOTANICAL NAME
Mimulus guttatus.

HABITAT
The banks of streams and rivers, and other wet places.

PLANT DESCRIPTION
A perennial, Mimulus grows to a height of about 1 foot (30 centimeters), with rounded, toothed, smooth leaves with several veins. It blooms from early to late summer, producing attractive yellow flowers.

REMEDY PREPARATION
Sun method.

INDICATIONS FOR USE
Specific, identifiable fears and anxieties. People in a negative Mimulus state tend to find the rough-and-tumble of life frightening, but usually keep their fears to themselves. They are frequently afraid of social contact, and so are prepared to go to great lengths to avoid it.

WHAT TREATMENT SHOULD ACHIEVE
Mimulus will help you to confront and deal with worries and anxieties, so enabling you to face the world with equanimity. It will also improve your understanding of others, particularly those with the same problems.

Environment
Look for Mimulus close to water, or in other damp places.

Single yellow flower

Rounded, toothed leaves

Hollow stem

BACH FLOWER REMEDIES

The Mimulus Remedy

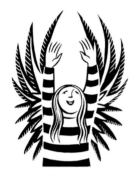

Liberating
Taking Mimulus will liberate you from oppressive fears, worries, and anxieties.

Most people have a particular worry or fear, which they would do almost anything to lose, particularly because they sometimes have to force themselves to try to overcome it. It could be something as simple as a fear of spiders, for instance, though it might well be something more serious than that. In such instances, Mimulus will help you, whatever your character type might be—and this is why most people take

the remedy. We have all been in the situation when we would give worlds for some form of secure relief and reassurance, which is what Mimulus, either on its own or in combination with other remedies, provides. If you are a Mimulus type, things may be more extreme, but the principle is still the same, provided that your fear or fears can be identified.

A plethora of choice

Obviously, a list of possible Mimulus fears has the potential to be almost endless, precisely because such identifiable fears are so common and everyday. They can range, from a fear of the dark going back to childhood to a fear of failing a crucial examination; or from a fear of being laid off in midcareer through no fault of one's own to running out of money when it comes to paying for health care in retirement.

It is a natural temptation not to face up to such problems, which is why people who suffer from them are sometimes reluctant to volunteer

information about what is worrying
them. It may be that they feel that
others may regard their fears as silly,
childish, or even selfish, so they try to
cover them up rather than face them
(though, in itself, this type of behavior
is also a fear that is recognizable). The
remedy helps them by reawakening
their innate courage, giving them
renewed faith in themselves.

What the Mimulus remedy helps
you to do is to get your life back on
track, so that you are able to take a
step back from what has been
worrying you, and see the problem
for what it really is. Remember, it all
comes down to your outlook on life,
which taking Mimulus can do a lot to
improve. You will become a more
confident, can-do sort of person, once
Mimulus has relieved what may well
be a passing mood.

The Negative State

The negative **Mimulus** state is characterized
by specific, identifiable fears or anxieties,
doubts, and fears.

Disaster signs
Even the smallest accident is a sign of a disaster waiting to happen in the negative Red Chestnut state.

RED CHESTNUT

This remedy helps you to deal with a very special type of fear, where, rather than worrying about yourself, you become obsessed about other people's well-being. Some people might call such fears altruistic, but nevertheless they should be confronted. Otherwise, if the worries become exaggerated, they may well become a burden not simply to you, but also to the people on whose behalf you are worrying. What the remedy does is to help you to be more constructive in the way you feel about other people, giving you the ability to remain completely calm if an actual emergency arises. This means that you will become a source of strength and reassurance, rather than, as Dr. Bach put it, "always fearing the worst, and always anticipating misfortune for others."

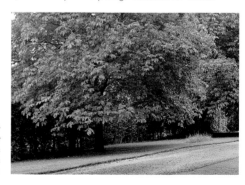

Environment
Look for Red Chestnut in parks, where its pinkish-red flowers make it easy to spot.

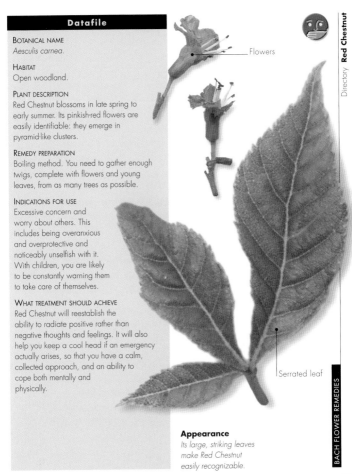

Datafile

BOTANICAL NAME
Aesculis carnea.

HABITAT
Open woodland.

PLANT DESCRIPTION
Red Chestnut blossoms in late spring to early summer. Its pinkish-red flowers are easily identifiable: they emerge in pyramid-like clusters.

REMEDY PREPARATION
Boiling method. You need to gather enough twigs, complete with flowers and young leaves, from as many trees as possible.

INDICATIONS FOR USE
Excessive concern and worry about others. This includes being overanxious and overprotective and noticeably unselfish with it. With children, you are likely to be constantly warning them to take care of themselves.

WHAT TREATMENT SHOULD ACHIEVE
Red Chestnut will reestablish the ability to radiate positive rather than negative thoughts and feelings. It will also help you keep a cool head if an emergency actually arises, so that you have a calm, collected approach, and an ability to cope both mentally and physically.

Flowers

Serrated leaf

Appearance
Its large, striking leaves make Red Chestnut easily recognizable.

The Red Chestnut Remedy

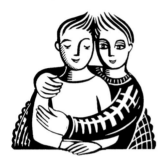

Overprotective
Being overprotective can produce opposite effects to the ones desired.

Red Chestnut is the ideal remedy "for those who find it difficult not to be anxious for other people." Dr. Bach noted additionally that sufferers from this form of fear had often "ceased to worry about themselves, but for those of whom they are fond they may suffer much, frequently anticipating that some unfortunate thing may happen to them." It is the kind of fear that manifests itself when, for instance, you gasp with a sharp intake of breath when you see someone starting to cross the road without looking, or if you see somebody missing their footing on a ladder. In the first instance, there is undoubtedly a car speeding around that corner, and, in the second, the slip is going to lead to a bone-breaking fall.

Looking for a remedy

It was actually a domestic mishap that inspired Dr. Bach to begin his quest for this remedy. What happened was recorded by Norah Weeks, Dr. Bach's closest colleague and, for many years after his death, one of the chief custodians of his teachings and traditions. Dr. Bach had had an accident with an ax while chopping wood, which "caused great anxiety on the part of those close to him as immediate first aid was applied to staunch the blood." When he had recovered, he commented that "we had experienced the state of mind of the next Remedy which he would seek." Because of his natural sensitivity, his colleagues' worrying had caused him to feel acute physical pain. Negative thoughts of this kind, he believed, could harm not only the people suffering from them but also their nearest and dearest.

Sometimes, such feelings are understandable. It is only natural to be apprehensive if, for example, your children have left home for the first time or if a partner is traveling long distances and has not been in touch for a while. It is less natural if such worries get out of proportion, so that you look only on the dark side, constantly anticipating some imminent disaster. The fussing and fretting that can result may be counterproductive, especially for children since overprotectiveness can damage their natural confidence.

As a rule, the Red Chestnut state is only temporary. The remedy can easily put matters to rights, though there are some true Red Chestnut types.

The Negative State

The negative **Red Chestnut** state is characterized by excessive concern and worry about others.

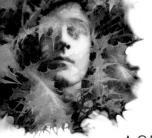

Anxiety
Aspen helps to overcome what psychologists term free-floating anxiety, caused by fears which arise for no apparent reason.

ASPEN

As opposed to Mimulus, which is the remedy for definable fears, Aspen is the remedy you take if you are suffering from what Dr. Bach described as "vague, unknown fears" for which there appears to be neither rhyme nor reason. These are what modern psychologists define as free-floating anxieties, which can vary in intensity up to and including full-blown terror and panic. Physical signs of this form of fear include sudden bouts of sweating, trembling and goosebumps, nightmares and sleeplessness. You may also suffer from groundless feelings of dread, which can strike suddenly with no clear, discernible focus. The remedy helps you by strengthening your ability to trust in yourself, the fear and apprehension lessening as your inner confidence recovers.

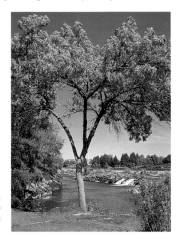

Harvesting
Aspen should be harvested before its leaf buds burst.

Datafile

BOTANICAL NAME
Populus tremula.

HABITAT
Woodland.

PLANT DESCRIPTION
Often referred to as the trembling tree because its leaves appear to flutter and shiver in the breeze, Aspen is a slender tree, seldom rising to more than 80 feet (24 meters) in height. Its female or male catkins appear in early to mid-spring, before the leaves, which are dark green, nearly circular, and wooly when young.

REMEDY PREPARATION
Boiling method. Gather twigs complete with male or female catkins and young leaf buds before the buds burst.

INDICATIONS FOR USE
Vague, groundless fears; sudden anxiety attacks with no apparent cause; and nightmares that make no sense when you try to interpret them.

WHAT TREATMENT SHOULD ACHIEVE
Taking Aspen will help you to reduce feelings of fear and apprehension. It will also help you to gain inner confidence, as you gradually become aware that there is something more meaningful and more positive to turn to, providing you with a firmer hold on reality.

Wooly leaf

Delicate
Aspen leaves and their stalks are so delicate that they will flutter in the slightest breeze.

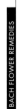

The Aspen Remedy

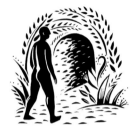

Courage
Taking Aspen will give you the courage to face the fear of the unknown.

Aspen fears are particularly terrifying precisely because, by definition, they are impossible to pin down. The thing that they all have in common is that their cause is unknown. In extreme cases, the problem becomes a vicious circle, from which it seems impossible to break free.

A severe state

Dr. Bach was quick to recognize the potential severity of the condition when he wrote that physical fears "are nothing compared to an unknown mental fear which comes over you like a cloud, bringing fear, terror, anxiety, and even panic without the slightest reason." Aspen fear may be associated with the sheer terror of the Rock Rose state, so both remedies are sometimes used together, especially if the emotional pressures are acute.

For Aspen people, almost every situation is full of hidden pitfalls. It seems as though they have a set of subconscious radar antennae that alert them to potential danger, so that they can react accordingly even before the danger actually arises. In contrast to the Mimulus state, where fears are clearly identifiable and so can be pinned down more easily, Aspen fears are always vague and indefinite and more difficult to deal with as a result. Dealing with the unknown is always more difficult than coming to terms with the finite.

People suffering from Aspen fear are often reluctant to talk through their problems, since, as they cannot pin down any definite reasons for them, they expect to be told that they are just imagining things, and have their fears and worries written off accordingly. If this happens, they naturally feel even worse than they did before.

Trembling with fear

The fear can be so strong that the entire body starts to tremble. Nervous tics may develop, together with bouts of sweating and fluttering sensations in the stomach. Successful treatment with the Aspen remedy, however, can lead to a complete transformation.

The remedy works by promoting self-confidence and self-belief, showing you not only that life is worth living, but also that you can gain awareness of what Dr. Bach termed "the great inner self in all of us which has the power to overcome all fears, all difficulties, all worries, all diseases." It also provides the knowledge that "the universal power of love stands behind all."

The Negative State

The negative **Aspen** state is characterized by vague, groundless fears that plague the mind and are of unknown origin.

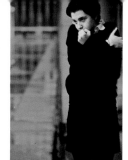

Extreme fear
Rock Rose fear can be so extreme that it may come close to paralyzing your will.

ROCK ROSE
Sometimes, fear can reach such a pitch that you find yourself absolutely incapable of dealing with it, accompanied by what can be likened to a form of mental paralysis as a result. By taking Rock Rose, you are reawakening your personal will, so that you can face up to what is terrorizing you, putting up a fight for what Dr. Bach termed "mental freedom." The remedy will assist you if you witness or are the victim of an accident, and you find yourself feeling great, overpowering fear, and unable to act or even think rationally. Rock Rose is one of the main ingredients in the emergency remedy combination sold as Rescue Remedy. In fact, Dr. Bach advised taking it "in all cases of urgency or danger," in combination with other remedies if advised.

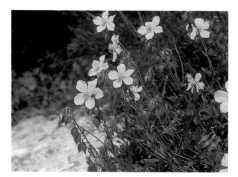

Environment
Rock Rose is a spreading shrub that is commonly found on chalky ground.

50

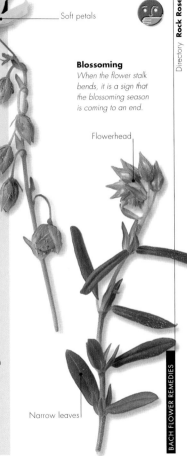

Soft petals

BOTANICAL NAME
Helianthemum nummularium.

HABITAT
Chalky, stony soils.

PLANT DESCRIPTION
A low, spreading, shrubby perennial, with small, bright yellow flowers that bloom in stages from early summer to early fall. Usually, only one or two flowers bloom at a time, the lower ones flowering before the upper ones. The full blossoming season is relatively short, the sign that it is coming to an end being when the flower stalks start to bend downward.

REMEDY PREPARATION
Sun method. Note that only wild Rock Rose should be used, not the multicolored cultivated equivalents.you may find growing in domestic rockeries.

INDICATIONS FOR USE
Extreme fear, terror, panic. These may not always be rational, but are nevertheless very real. Also, if you are haunted by bad dreams, nightmares, and hallucinations, or suffer from suddenly escalating anxieties when faced with either physical or mental emergencies.

WHAT TREATMENT SHOULD ACHIEVE
Rock Rose was described by Dr. Bach as the remedy "of emergency" and it acts quickly to bring about positive results. To liberate you from your fears, it boosts your reserves of nervous energy and stimulates the inner reserve of courage you normally possess, encouraging a swing in mood from a strongly negative to a strongly positive state.

Blossoming
When the flower stalk bends, it is a sign that the blossoming season is coming to an end.

Flowerhead

Narrow leaves

The Rock Rose Remedy

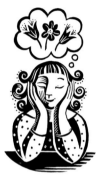

Panic attacks
Rock Rose will calm the panic attacks that can arise as a result of deep fear.

Rock Rose stimulates your internal reserves of courage and steadfastness, which is why Dr. Bach recommended its use in all "cases of emergency." Later, he was to choose it as one of the most important components of Rescue Remedy (see pages 214–217). Even on its own, however, Dr. Bach noted that "many an alarming case has been better within minutes or hours of it being given."

Sip two drops in a glass of water or place a few drops on the tongue. If you are in a negative Rock Rose state, any emergency you feel you are facing is very real to you, even if, to an outside observer the particular set of circumstances does not appear to be quite as life-threatening or menacing as you sense it to be.

Facing the problem

It is as if you personally are under siege and there is no prospect of a relieving army coming to rescue you. It is as if everything that is happening to you is quickly taking you in completely the opposite direction to the one you want to be going in. The fears themselves can feel just like a sudden kick in the stomach and seem impossible to escape from or resolve. At its worst, you may find it impossible to come to terms or deal with all the unpleasant things you believe are facing you.

Luckily, in most cases, the problems that give rise to extreme Rock Rose fears are, in themselves, only temporary. This is especially true of children suffering from bad dreams, when the advice is to give them sips of the remedy until their fears subside. Even more fortunately, there is no such thing as a Rock Rose type—the remedy is purely a mood remedy. It quickly sets things right, so that, whatever the problem behind the fear, you can deal with it.

Dr. Bach also recommended taking the remedy if "the condition is so serious as to cause intense fear to those around you." Whatever the situation, taking the remedy should transform matters. By helping to mobilize your internal reserves of courage, it will give you the strength to grow beyond your fears and to deal with them accordingly. You have the reassurance of Dr. Bach's words that "from being full of terror and in a state of panic, you will become a picture of calm, serene courage."

The Negative State

The negative **Rock Rose** state is characterized by overwhelming fears and terrors when situations feel like emergencies.

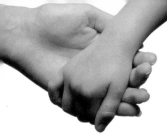

Loss of control
Cherry Plum provides a helping hand for those who fear they will lose control of themselves.

CHERRY PLUM

The most suitable remedy for helping people who are afraid of the damage they can cause themselves and, indeed, others, if they lose control of themselves and their actions, is Cherry Plum. It should be taken if you feel as if an inner time bomb is ticking away, which, if it explodes, will make you do something terrible against your will. The danger is the risk of becoming enslaved to the destructive urges that arise as a result of the emotional stress, although you are only too aware of the negative consequences of submitting to them. The remedy acts to defuse the situation, and the associated emotional traumas that can arise as a result of it. It gives you the courage to deal with the crisis you are facing by confronting and resolving what is causing it.

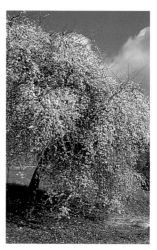

Harvesting
Cherry Plum blooms in early spring. The blossoms should be gathered before the leaves appear.

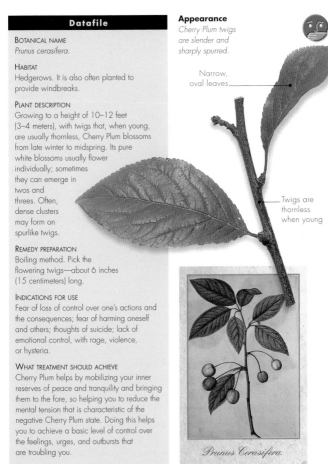

Datafile

BOTANICAL NAME
Prunus cerasifera.

HABITAT
Hedgerows. It is also often planted to provide windbreaks.

PLANT DESCRIPTION
Growing to a height of 10–12 feet (3–4 meters), with twigs that, when young, are usually thornless, Cherry Plum blossoms from late winter to midspring. Its pure white blossoms usually flower individually; sometimes they can emerge in twos and threes. Often, dense clusters may form on spurlike twigs.

REMEDY PREPARATION
Boiling method. Pick the flowering twigs—about 6 inches (15 centimeters) long.

INDICATIONS FOR USE
Fear of loss of control over one's actions and the consequences; fear of harming oneself and others; thoughts of suicide; lack of emotional control, with rage, violence, or hysteria.

WHAT TREATMENT SHOULD ACHIEVE
Cherry Plum helps by mobilizing your inner reserves of peace and tranquility and bringing them to the fore, so helping you to reduce the mental tension that is characteristic of the negative Cherry Plum state. Doing this helps you to achieve a basic level of control over the feelings, urges, and outbursts that are troubling you.

Appearance
Cherry Plum twigs are slender and sharply spurred.

Narrow, oval leaves

Twigs are thornless when young

Prunus Cerasifera.

The Cherry Plum Remedy

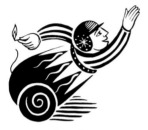

Control
*Cherry Plum helps to
release negative thoughts
without losing control.*

Cherry Plum is the remedy that
Dr. Bach devised to help to
overcome fear of loss of reason
and self-control. It is an extreme state of
mind, as a result of which you may feel
that you are heading for an actual
mental breakdown.

It is almost as if you can mentally and
physically feel destructive forces welling
up deep within you: your inability to
deal with them causes you to worry that
you may injure yourself or, indeed, do
harm to others. In extreme desperation,
some sufferers even contemplate suicide
to escape from the deep depression

that is the result of being trapped in
such a desperate emotional state.
Unaided, there appears to be no other
way out of the intense suffering that you
are being caused, so that you may fear
that you will kill yourself as a way out.

Giving up the fight

Spiritually and mentally, the fear can
become so intense that you can get to
the point when you simply want to give
up the unequal struggle against the ever
more powerful forces that seem to be
gaining control within you and over
you. The natural consequence of this
state of affairs is an increase in the fear
level, while any attempts you may be
making to keep your fears suppressed
seem more and more unavailing. Fear
of the frustrated rage that may follow is
yet another problem.

If you are a parent, for instance, you
may worry that you may actually hit
your children; it is tempting to strike out
in all directions, particularly at those
you love, regardless of the potentially
hurtful consequences.

Even if things have not reached such an impasse, there is no doubt that the remedy will help you to recover and dig yourself out of the pit into which you have fallen. The Cherry Plum remedy, according to Dr. Bach, drives away "all the wrong ideas" and gives sufferers "mental strength and confidence." The crisis can now be seen to have a positive side. It gives you the opportunity to learn and move on with your life.

The remedy works by helping you to confront your worst nightmares and deal with all the negative emotions your fears represent. You will find yourself connected to an enormous reservoir of strength that will help to guide you through all your problems. The bonus is that, by exploring your feelings, you can come to terms with whatever triggered the fears.

The Negative State

The negative **Cherry Plum** state is characterized by the fear of a loss of reason and self-control.

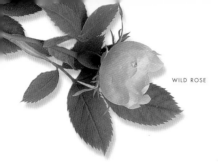

WILD ROSE

REMEDIES IN ACTION
Dr. Bach believed that the amazing herbal remedies he had discovered should be freely available so that the widest possible audience could share in their benefits. Similarly, he was an advocate of self-treatment whenever practical: the truly successful Bach practitioner has no patients left: all are fully equipped to treat themselves. The case studies here demonstrate a selection of the Bach flower remedies in action.

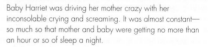

Case Study

Baby Harriet was driving her mother crazy with her inconsolable crying and screaming. It was almost constant—so much so that mother and baby were getting no more than an hour or so of sleep a night.

Both Harriet and her mother were advised to take **Olive** to help them deal with their mutual exhaustion. In addition, Harriet was prescribed **Impatiens** and **Cherry Plum**.

Within a week of taking the remedies, Harriet had settled into a regular sleeping pattern, and although she still cried occasionally, the screaming had stopped completely.

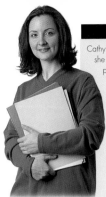

Case Study

Cathy was tense and anxious about her work, looking nervous although she tried to smile and laugh all the time. She constantly felt under pressure, physically exhausted, and unable to cope. She had been diagnosed as suffering from clinical depression. Fear of missing deadlines was uppermost in her mind, but she was finding it hard to keep motivated.

Agrimony was prescribed as Cathy's type remedy, together with **Elm** to help her come to terms with her responsibilities, **White Chestnut** to calm her thoughts, **Mustard** for her depression, **Larch** for her lack of confidence, and **Olive** for her physical tiredness. **Rescue Remedy** and **Clematis** were also suggested. After just a week, there was an obvious change. Cathy's confidence had started to return and she had new energy and enthusiasm.

Case Study

Peter was an impatient, energetic, fast-moving businessman. He had started complaining of frequent headaches and continuously catching colds from his work colleagues. He was happy working long hours, but basically he felt under a lot of pressure.

Peter seemed to be an **Impatiens** type, so this remedy was advised to help him to slow down and relax. He also needed **Oak** to stop him from pushing himself so hard.

Vine was prescribed to discourage him from trying to dominate others and to encourage him to rely on his positive powers of natural leadership.

Finally, **Olive** was added as a tonic to help him recharge his batteries.

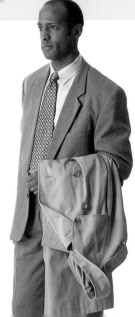

Remedies for Uncertainty

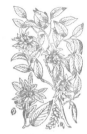

Decisive
Hornbeam combats mental tiredness and allows you to get the job done.

Uncertainty and indecision affect everyone from time to time. Even Dr. Bach, so it is recorded, experienced their negative effects as he embarked on his search for remedies to counter their varied aspects. Eventually, what he discovered was that there were six distinct uncertainty remedies in all, each with their own individual properties and uses.

Cerato, for instance, helps you if you find yourself doubting the validity of your own decisions through a lack of self-confidence. Things may reach such a pitch that you find it impossible to stand up for yourself and your opinions. Instead, you constantly tend to seek others' advice as to what you should do and whether or not you are doing the right thing. Scleranthus, in contrast, is the remedy to try if you are so indecisive that you are are unable to take any decisions at all. It helps you to summon up the initiative to cut through all the uncertainties that are besetting you, and to stop prevaricating and sitting on the fence. This enables you to start being positive, take and make decisions and stick to them.

Dealing with discouragement

Gentian will help you to deal with the despondency and discouragement that can result from a disappointment or setback by giving you the courage and confidence that you need to try again. If, however, the negative feelings snowball, Gorse is the remedy of choice, since it will help to relieve the feelings of pessimism and despondency that will otherwise come to dominate you. This state is not always that easy to distinguish from the Wild Rose state. The basic difference is that Gorse people can usually be persuaded to at least try something new, while Wild Rose types are trapped in apathy.

Hornbeam will help you if you are finding it impossible to get down to things. Wild Oat, in contrast, will help you if you feel frustrated by what you are doing, since all your inner feelings are telling you that, even if you are successful, you are not fulfilling yourself because, for whatever reason, you are not taking your true path in life. The remedy helps you to deal with the consequent uncertainty that such a realization naturally causes by giving you the ability you need to take a more rational, balanced view.

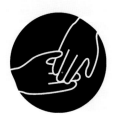

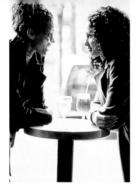

Reassurance
People in a negative Cerato state are only too prone to seeking out others for constant reassurance rather than making their own decisions.

CERATO
The odd one out among the Bach flower remedies, Cerato is the only one made from cultivated plants. In northern climes, it does not grow in the wild and, to survive, needs to be protected against frost during the winter. Cerato will help if you lack faith in your own judgment when it comes to making decisions. Instead, you are constantly seeking the advice of others, since you believe that they always know what's what better than you do. This means that you may well be getting on the nerves of friends and family through your constant questioning and demands for reassurance. The remedy gives you the confidence to think for yourself and to accept that what you decide for yourself is right for you.

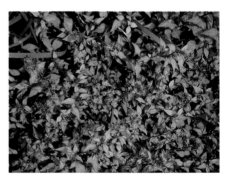

Origin
Cerato is a shrub that originally came from the Himalayas.

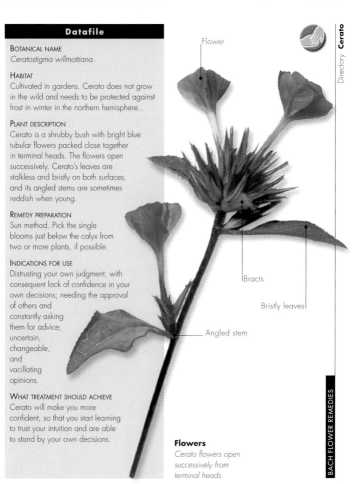

Datafile

BOTANICAL NAME
Ceratostigma willmottiana.

HABITAT
Cultivated in gardens. Cerato does not grow in the wild and needs to be protected against frost in winter in the northern hemisphere..

PLANT DESCRIPTION
Cerato is a shrubby bush with bright blue tubular flowers packed close together in terminal heads. The flowers open successively. Cerato's leaves are stalkless and bristly on both surfaces, and its angled stems are sometimes reddish when young.

REMEDY PREPARATION
Sun method. Pick the single blooms just below the calyx from two or more plants, if possible.

INDICATIONS FOR USE
Distrusting your own judgment, with consequent lack of confidence in your own decisions; needing the approval of others and constantly asking them for advice; uncertain, changeable, and vacillating opinions.

WHAT TREATMENT SHOULD ACHIEVE
Cerato will make you more confident, so that you start learning to trust your intuition and are able to stand by your own decisions.

Flower

Bracts

Bristly leaves

Angled stem

Flowers
Cerato flowers open successively from terminal heads.

The Cerato Remedy

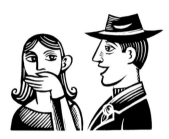

Alienating
*The demands you make on others
to help you make decisions may
serve only to alienate them.*

If you are a Cerato type, you suffer from the inability to trust in your own judgements and are always questioning your own decisions as a result. For this reason, you constantly seek advice from others, which may well get on their nerves as your demands on their tolerance constantly increase. In fact, you may well find that you are making the wrong choices through relying on their advice.

If you need this remedy you know in your heart what you want to do. You have made your decision. But as soon as you go to act, doubt creeps in and you feel the need to look for reassurance. You are certain that you know what to do, but you don't trust yourself and think other people will be better at taking decisions than you are.

Gaining wisdom

This is where the Cerato remedy comes into its own. Taking it gives you not only the ability to decide on appropriate courses of action but also, even more importantly, the boost in self-confidence you need to have the courage of your convictions to put what you decide to do into practice.

Without the remedy, on the other hand, the chances are that you will continue to mistrust your intuitions and, instead of taking heed of them, find yourself relying more and more on outside advice to make up your mind for you. Equally, it means that all the information and knowledge that you are undoubtedly getting from the people you are consulting is not being put to any good use, since the negative

Cerato state means that you find yourself to be incapable of learning from it, or being guided by it.

Renewing your confidence

To overcome the lack of confidence that lies at the heart of the problem, Cerato works to make the guiding inner voices that you have been suppressing come to the fore again. The more you put your trust in them and what they are telling you, the more clearly they will guide you along the path to an appropriate decision. The real breakthrough comes when you find that you are empowered to make rapid decisions with a previously unknown degree of certainty. Rather than appearing gullible or even stupid, you will find yourself once again enthusiastic, curious, and eager to learn.

The Negative State

The negative **Cerato** state is characterized by a lack of trust and confidence in your own judgements and decisions.

Balancing act

Taking Scleranthus will stop you from balancing on a tightrope of indecision and help you to bring things to a point.

SCLERANTHUS

If you suffer from a chronic inability to take any decision, however small, with the consequence that you find yourself in a dilemma, sitting on the fence whenever a choice has to be made, Scleranthus should be able to help you. Not only will it help to relieve what can be a painful mental trauma, it will also help you to focus your thoughts, so that you can assess your options more clearly and come to trust in your own powers of decision. It can also help you to cope with mood swings and consequent emotional imbalances, especially if your moods are rapidly changing. As a result of your newfound decisiveness and belief in your ability to trust in and implement your decisions, you will gain an invaluable feeling of inner stability and consequent peace of mind.

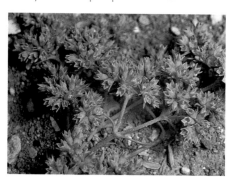

Appearance

Scleranthus is small and bushy, with tiny, awl-shaped leaves.

Datafile

BOTANICAL NAME
Scleranthus annuus.

HABITAT
Sandy and gravelly soils.

PLANT DESCRIPTION
Scleranthus is a bushy annual with pale or dark green flowers. These can be difficult to find because they blend in with their background so perfectly. They bloom from midsummer to early fall, growing in clusters, either in the forks of the stems or in terminal tufts.

REMEDY PREPARATION
Sun method.

INDICATIONS FOR USE
Inability to make decisions; dithering between one option and another; insecurity; inability to trust in personal judgment; extreme mood fluctuations; grasshopper mind.

WHAT TREATMENT SHOULD ACHIEVE
Scleranthus encourages decisiveness, enabling you to cut through this type of uncertainty and make calm, precise choices and judgements. As a result of taking it, your powers of concentration and determination will be increased and you should find yourself becoming mentally more flexible and versatile as a result.

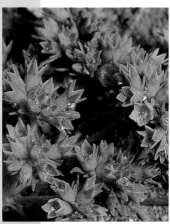

Color variation
When they emerge, the color of the flowers varies depending on the nature of the soil.

The Scleranthus Remedy

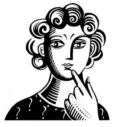

Indecision
*If you are incapable
of making up your mind,
Scleranthus can help.*

Scleranthus, according to Dr. Bach, is the remedy that will be most helpful to "those who find it difficult to decide what they want and to make up their minds about what they would like. They try first one thing, and then another. They feel they want two or three things at the same time, but cannot decide which." When faced with a choice, Scleranthus type people do not know what to do; a classic sign of this kind of personality is a constantly changing mind. Over a long period of time, this sort of dilemma of indecision causes them to gradually withdraw into themselves and bottle up their emotional problems. They would rather struggle on on their own, rather than, as a Cerato person would do, seek advice from others to help them in their decision making and taking.

Scleranthus, however, will help you to deal with more than just the inability to make or take decisions. It will also help you to treat the other physical symptoms associated with the type, which may seem to come and go, just like your wishes and desires. If you have a temperature, for instance, it may swing up and down and back and forth, with no obvious pattern.

Mood swings and changes

Other characteristics of Scleranthus people may include rapid mood swings – from cheerful to depressed, for instance – and, in conversation, there may be a tendency to jump suddenly from one topic to another. Someone who finds it impossible to decide what to eat in a restaurant, or a woman unable to decide between two boyfriends, are both classic Scleranthus cases. Many people in need of Scleranthus remedy change their clothes several times a day as a reaction to their fluctuating moods.

Combining remedies

As with the other remedies Dr. Bach discovered, however, it is sometimes the case that more than one remedy is needed. If you feel that there are associated problems, you need to identify what they are and the remedies that are appropriate for them. In such a situation, though, you should always bear in mind the importance of starting by treating current states of mind, rather than harking back to past ones. This means that you should certainly consider taking extra remedies if these are also needed to treat your problems.

The Negative State

The negative **Scleranthus** state is characterized by indecision and an inability to make up your own mind.

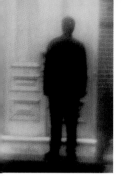

Obstacle course
Gentian enables you to combat doubt and discouragement and to overcome all obstacles in your path.

GENTIAN
If you become discouraged easily and knocked off your stride, feeling that even the slightest things seem to be going against you, Gentian is the remedy to employ. It differs from Mustard, which Dr. Bach also advised using to raise the spirits, because, in the case of Gentian, the problems triggering the depression stem from a known, rather than an unknown, cause. Sinking easily into despondency and giving up easily even on things that you feel you merit, such as recognition for work well done, are symptoms of a negative Gentian state. The remedy works by helping you to dispel the negative states of mind that are plaguing you, giving you the ability to stick to your guns, and remain true to your goals.

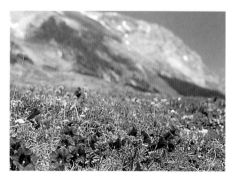

Environment
Gentian favors a dry, hillside habitat.

Datafile

BOTANICAL NAME
Gentiana amarella.

HABITAT
Dry hilly pastures, cliffs, and dunes.

PLANT DESCRIPTION
The plant is a biennial that grows
to a height of about 8 inches
(20 centimeters). Its deep purplish-blue
flowers, which grow either individually
or in clusters on upright stems in the
axils of the leaves, blossom from late
summer to midfall. The leaves are dark
green and marked with three
prominent veins.

REMEDY PREPARATION
Sun method. Gather the flowers just
below the calyx.

INDICATIONS FOR USE
Easily becoming discouraged by even
a minor setback or failure; uncertainty
due to lack of faith and confidence.

WHAT TREATMENT SHOULD ACHIEVE
Gentian encourages optimism,
preventing you from being influenced
adversely by what has happened to
you in the past, or by past events that
are casting their shadows over the present.
By enhancing your inner confidence, it gives
you the assurance you need to believe that
problems can be overcome and that,
ultimately, you will be successful in whatever
you undertake.

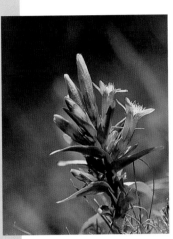

Flowers
The flowers grow on
stalks in the axils of the
plant's dark leaves.

The Gentian Remedy

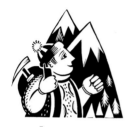

Encouragement
Gentian enables you to take heart and renew your efforts.

Gentian will help you if you are prone to feelings of doubt and despondency, since every obstacle in life that comes your way, however minor, starts to seem insurmountable. Classic signs that you may need the remedy are if you feel you have lost your drive and are somehow lacking the determination to carry on, especially when confronted with the fact that things are not going precisely according to plan. If this happens, it may take only a seemingly insignificant incident to rattle your confidence—what you need in these circumstances is help to regain your ability to get things in balance and reestablish a due sense of proportion. Without taking steps to achieve this, things may go from bad to worse.

In such situations, rather than gritting your teeth and getting on with things in the belief that it is more likely than not that things will turn out for the best after all, your response, though perfectly understandable, is completely the opposite. Instead of rising to the challenge, you become discouraged and dejected.

Doubts and fears

More than this—your doubts constantly gnaw away at you to lower your morale still further, making matters even worse. As a result, you may find yourself increasingly unable to cope with the problems and disappointments that life naturally brings.

In order for the Gentian remedy to work for you, you should be able to identify the circumstances that are triggering your despondency and discouragement. This is the essential first step on the road to recovering the positive approach to life and its problems that, underneath it all, you still possess. Classic examples of the types of problem that may affect you include a setback on the road to recovery during convalescence, or the failure to get a promotion you expected. What you need is to recover the ability to see such things for what they are—challenges that can be overcome with a little determined effort.

In many cases, the problem may be only temporary, but sometimes things can be compounded, as self-doubt and heavy-heartedness reach such a pitch that a state of perpetual pessimism and persistent doubt takes over and you fall into a Gorse state.

To avoid this—(see pages 74–77)—prompt treatment with the Gentian remedy is important.

The Negative State

The negative **Gentian** state is characterized by feelings of doubt and despair, and being faced with insurmountable obstacles.

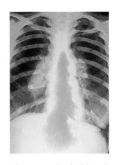

GORSE

Bach practitioners often describe the Gorse state as being a step further downhill from the Gentian one (see pages 70–73). Sometimes, this can take hold with little or no warning, with discouragement degenerating all too suddenly into despair and utter hopelessness. If Gentian people feel like giving up when things start getting difficult or problematical, Gorse people really do just that, sinking into a state of abject pessimism and utter hopelessness from which they find it impossible to extract themselves. This remains the case even when there are other people around to help them by suggesting possible solutions to their plight. Gorse remedy, however, encourages a sense of optimism and purpose, triggering the renewal of hope that people in this state lack.

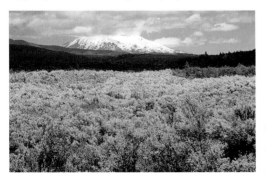

Environment
Gorse is an evergreen shrub that is particularly common on heaths.

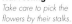

Datafile

BOTANICAL NAME
Ulex europaeus.

HABITAT
Dry, exposed commons and heaths, stony soil.

PLANT DESCRIPTION
Gorse is a bushy evergreen with abundant golden-yellow flowers. These are at their best in early to mid-spring, although, if the weather is mild, flowering may start earlier than this. The flowers grow individually from the leaf axils of the previous year's shoots. The leaves start off soft and hairy, but, by the time they have reached maturity, they have developed into sharply pointed green spikes.

REMEDY PREPARATION
Sun method (midspring to early summer). Choose big clumps of flowers, picking them by their stalks.

INDICATIONS FOR USE
Deep depression after something goes wrong; ongoing despair; abject pessimism and no hope for a better future.

WHAT TREATMENT SHOULD ACHIEVE
Gorse restores belief, giving you the desire to regain a natural emotional equilibrium. By lifting you out of your gloom, it will help you to gain in self-awareness and self-respect, sharpening your sense of pride in who you are, and what you are able to accomplish.

Harvesting
Take care to pick the flowers by their stalks.

Flowers on leaf axils

Leaf spurs

The Gorse Remedy

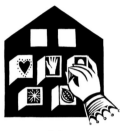

Optimism
*Gorse helps you to realize that
life is worth living after all.*

Dr. Bach counted Gorse as one of his original seven "helpers"—herbs that paved the way for healing, especially in cases of long-established, chronic illness and disease. Many people in the negative Gorse state have suffered, or are suffering, from such complaints. No form of medical treatment has brought about a total cure, so they have come to the end of the road mentally, having given up hope, convincing themselves that their problems cannot be resolved. Although they can still be persuaded to undertake treatment—this is the key difference between the Gorse and the Wild Rose states of mind—they are nevertheless sure that nothing that may be suggested will do anything to help, or improve the situation in which they find themselves. In such cases, leaving things as they are will be counterproductive, since the existence of such negative expectations simply reinforces the hold the disease has on them.

In the Bach system of healing, Gorse embodies the quality of hope—and this is precisely what it gives back to you, so that you feel there is a point to life once again. According to Dr. Bach, the remedy is for those who have lost the heart to try any more. They look, he said, as though "they needed more sunshine in their lives to drive away the clouds."

Renewing hope

This is exactly what the remedy helps to provide. It renews your sense of hope and encourages you in the belief that all is not lost and that there are things worth looking forward to in the future.

What it also dispels is the dark cloud of apathy that seems to have fallen completely over you. Taking the remedy quickly will help to unleash all the hidden reserves of strength and courage that still lie deep inside you. As a result, you will be able to take heart once again and be prepared to give life another try. This is not to say that the problems that have triggered the condition will necessarily vanish, but you will be in a far better state to deal with them and cope with whatever the consequences may be.

This particularly applies if, like many Gorse people, you are a martyr to chronic illness, which keeps on recurring. In such instances, the profound change the remedy can bring about is often the initial spark that the body and its immune system need to jump-start the natural healing process.

The Negative State

The negative **Gorse** state is characterized by utter hopelessness and despair especially after a chronic illness or disease.

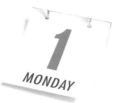

MONDAY

Monday blues
Because a sign of a negative Hornbeam state is the inability to face work, it is often termed the Monday morning remedy.

HORNBEAM

When you feel exhausted mentally and physically at the mere thought of how much work you have to do, taking Hornbeam will help you to overcome the problem. You should also take it when you find yourself putting off starting a job or task, since it also counters procrastination. By strengthening your determination, it gives you that little extra push you need to settle down to things and get started. Once you have given the remedy a chance to work, you will find that all your feelings of weariness melt away by themselves and that the task in hand can be completed without difficulty.

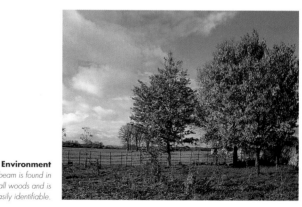

Environment
Hornbeam is found in small woods and is easily identifiable.

Datafile

BOTANICAL NAME
Carpinus betulus.

HABITAT
Woods and coppices.

PLANT DESCRIPTION·
Hornbeam has smooth, light gray bark and a deeply fluted trunk. Male and female flowers grow together on the same tree, blossoming in mid- to late spring. The males—drooping, cylindrical, sharp-tipped catkins—grow in the axils of the previous year's leaves; the females—produced in pairs, facing each other, at the end of short lateral shoots—stand erect until the fruit forms, when they hang down.

REMEDY PREPARATION
Boiling method. Pick young twigs, with leaves and both male and female flowers.

INDICATIONS FOR USE
Feeling that you lack the strength to fulfill your daily tasks; procrastinating; feeling heavy-headed, tired, and deprived of vigor; getting up in the morning more tired than when you went to bed.

WHAT TREATMENT SHOULD ACHIEVE
Hornbeam stimulates the mind and ensures that you have a clear, cool head. By boosting -confidence in your strength, it will help you to master any task that lies ahead, even if, at first sight, it appears to be beyond your powers.

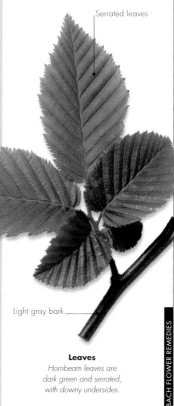

Serrated leaves

Light gray bark

Leaves
Hornbeam leaves are dark green and serrated, with downy undersides.

The Hornbeam Remedy

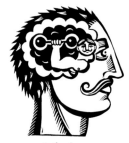

Enthusiasm
Hornbeam helps you to overcome mental tiredness and fatigue.

Often jokingly referred to as the "Monday morning remedy," Hornbeam fulfills various functions in the Bach system of healing. It was one of the remedies Dr. Bach discovered in that great burst of creative energy that particularly characterized the last years of his life, as he responded to the challenge of filling the remaining gaps he perceived existed in his system and fulfilled his dream of making it totally complete.

Basically, the remedy will help you if, to paraphrase Dr. Bach's own description, you are convinced that you lack the mental or physical strength to bear the burdens that life is placing on you (although, strictly speaking, the fatigue is illusory and more to do with the mind than the body). When you suffer from this fatigue, even routine, everyday matters seem too much to cope with, but, when you buckle down, you generally succeed in meeting your obligations. The remedy will also help you if you believe that some part of the mind or body needs to be strengthened or reinforced before you can focus on fulfilling your tasks and responsibilities successfully.

Short term and long term

Often, the Hornbeam state is short-lived. Longer-term Hornbeam weariness, however, can occur if everything starts to seem like a tiresome duty, rather than something that you can approach positively and get pleasure from tackling successfully. Such weariness can vanish instantly, however, when something out of the ordinary happens, giving you the opportunity to make a clean break with routine. This happens to all of us from time to time. No matter how conscientious and dedicated we are, there is nothing like a new challenge to stimulate what sometimes may be a flagging interest.

If you are in a negative Hornbeam state, the remedy acts as a tonic, which will help you to recover your *joie de vivre*. Both your work and life itself will become a pleasure again, as you regain your energy and enthusiasm. Your emotional strength will be restored, as you receive that all-important boost that will help to ensure your future success.

You should note that Dr. Bach devised another remedy—Olive—to help people to cope with tiredness resulting from overwork. This is a totally different emotional state (see pages 104–105) and should be treated as such.

The Negative State

The negative **Hornbeam** state is characterized by a lack of physical and mental strength, especially mental fatigue.

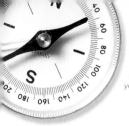

WILD OAT

What Dr. Bach called his Wild Oat remedy actually comes from a wild grass that is noted for its short flowering time. It was discovered just after Dr. Bach moved to Oxfordshire, completing the first series of 19 remedies. One of the specific times that Wild Oat is particularly advised is if you are feeling frustrated and dissatisfied as a result of your inability to find your true path and direction in life. You know that you have reached a crossroad, but you do not know which way to turn for the best. The remedy helps by encouraging you to listen to your guiding inner voice, so that you can establish what you really want in life and in which direction you need to be heading. It points you to fulfilling yourself and your vocation.

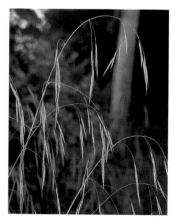

Description
What Dr. Bach called Wild Oat is, in fact, Wood or Hairy Brome.

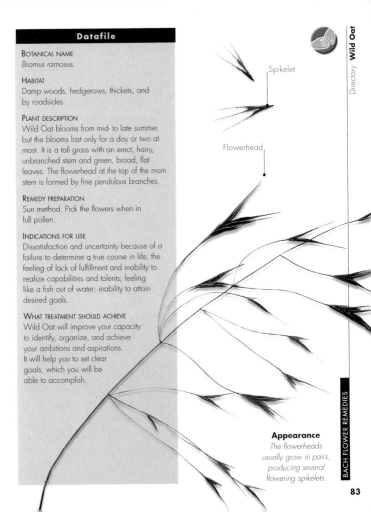

Datafile

BOTANICAL NAME
Bromus ramosus.

HABITAT
Damp woods, hedgerows, thickets, and by roadsides.

PLANT DESCRIPTION
Wild Oat blooms from mid- to late summer, but the blooms last only for a day or two at most. It is a tall grass with an erect, hairy, unbranched stem and green, broad, flat leaves. The flowerhead at the top of the main stem is formed by fine pendulous branches.

REMEDY PREPARATION
Sun method. Pick the flowers when in full pollen.

INDICATIONS FOR USE
Dissatisfaction and uncertainty because of a failure to determine a true course in life; the feeling of lack of fulfillment and inability to realize capabilities and talents; feeling like a fish out of water; inability to attain desired goals.

WHAT TREATMENT SHOULD ACHIEVE
Wild Oat will improve your capacity to identify, organize, and achieve your ambitions and aspirations. It will help you to set clear goals, which you will be able to accomplish.

Spikelet

Flowerhead

Appearance
The flowerheads usually grow in pairs, producing several flowering spikelets.

The Wild Oat Remedy

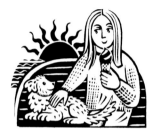

Purpose
*Wild Oat will help
if you are unsure of your
purpose in life.*

Wild Oat is bound up with the twinned qualities of vocation and purposefulness. If you are in a negative Wild Oat state, you will have failed to identify your true vocation and will feel dissatisfied and unfulfilled.

This is even more of a pity than usual, since, typically, Wild Oat people are blessed with many talents. In fact, it could be argued that they run the risk of being spoiled for choice. Life, it seems, is perpetually offering them new opportunities and chances to shine, but because they lack the real inner certainty that will allow them to make a final, definitive choice, they are prone to following false trails. Ultimately, when these prove unsatisfactory, they may well abandon or even tear down everything they have built up in the hope that, by making a completely fresh start, they will end up with something that will be far more satisfactory. They may also feel that life is passing them by, despite all their undoubted talents.

Fulfilling yourself

Occasionally, too, there may be a discrepancy between scale of aspiration and level of ability, with the result that you find it difficult to bridge the gap between the two. This can happen, for instance, if you have set your sights on something that you know, in your heart, you are unqualified to do. If so, it can prove hard to fulfill yourself and you may feel constantly frustrated.

If you start to take Wild Oat, you will gradually feel yourself growing calmer, clearer, and more certain in mind, body, and spirit. Little by little, a more precise picture of what you really want will emerge and you will start to act intuitively, rather than on impulse. Life will now be much more fulfilling. You will be able to recognize your potential and to develop it; you will know how to prioritize your ambitions and not allow yourself to be deflected from them; and you will find you can do far more than you imagined possible.

By finally deciding on a specific course of action and accepting inner guidance, you will achieve a more balanced perspective on the world and your place within it. As a result, the life you live will be filled with usefulness and happiness. You will have established just what you want to do in your life and what you want to accomplish with it, and will not allow interference with that decision.

The Negative State

The negative **Wild Oat** state is characterized by a deep dissatisfaction with life combined with a lack of fulfillment.

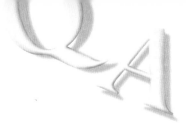

QUESTIONS & ANSWERS
Decades after Dr. Bach's death in 1936, more people than ever before are taking his healing remedies, which are still prepared in the way he specified. Bach practitioners all over the world still teach Dr. Bach's clear, simple precepts. Here are some of the most frequently asked questions about the remedies, answered by the experts at the Bach Centre.

Q My toddler is only two years old. Can I give him Rescue Remedy if the situation calls for it, and what type of situation would this be? How much of it should I give?

A *Children can become ill very quickly and you should always contact your doctor if your child becomes unwell. In less serious situations,* *Rescue Remedy can be given when your child is feeling delicate. Put four drops into a little cooled boiled water and mix with their food, or give it by teaspoon. It is not possible to overdose (though the remedy should always be diluted), nor are there any side effects. It is not habit-forming.*

Q Could you tell me if the Bach remedies are safe for children? Are there any that are unsafe?

A *All of the remedies are entirely safe, even for newborn babies. The only thing to remember is that, because they are preserved in alcohol, they should be diluted before use. The instructions will be on the bottle.*

Q I would like to know whether Rescue Remedy is effective in calming panic attacks for people who are unable to take remedies such as Prozac. Also, are there any side effects? Can Rescue Remedy be taken with blood pressure medication or any other prescribed medicine?

A *Rescue Remedy is natural and safe and will not react with the other medication you mention. The only possible contraindication is due to the fact that it is preserved in brandy, so if there are any reasons that you cannot take a minute quantity of alcohol, you need to check with the person who has prescribed your other medication.*

Q Recently, my girlfriend consulted an alternative practitioner, who asked her to hold her hand over preparations of the 38 Bach flowers. After this she was told that she needed to take Scleranthus and Clematis, since she was dreamy, prone to fainting, not in touch with reality, and almost suicidal. My question is that to make any such diagnosis, oughtn't there to have been be an interview first? This never happened. Am I right?

A *There are people who select remedies in the way you describe, but the way Dr. Bach used to work is to listen to what someone has to say, ask questions, and select remedies based on how the person feels. No occult methods are necessary—and they often fail to work anyway.*

Q My friend will not consume any alcohol. How can he apply the remedies?

A *Putting the drops on the wrist or other pulse points will be effective. Using a vaporizer may also work, but will not be as immediately effective.*

Q I am 26 weeks pregnant and feel very stressed. Which remedies would you suggest?

A *Try Rescue Remedy to help you to cope with the stress. Put four drops into a glass of water and sip it until you feel calmer as often as you need to.*

Remedies for Lack of Interest in Present Circumstances

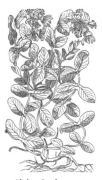

Living in the past
Honeysuckle helps if you are always looking back to past times, not to present ones.

Insufficient interest in present circumstances, Dr. Bach said, fell into seven different types, for each of which he devised an remedy. To help people with a tendency to live in their dreams rather than facing up to reality, he advised Clematis. Such people are often creative and artistic, but seem to live in a world of their own. They are likely to drop off to sleep at odd moments, but are equally prone to building castles in the air, making plans that are somehow never realized.

Excessive nostalgia

For people who feel that all their happiness lies behind them, Dr. Bach recommended Honeysuckle for its ability to focus the mind on the present and put the past into perspective. It can be a particularly effective remedy at times of bereavement, when it should be combined with Star of Bethlehem to help to counter grief, sorrow, and shock. Wild Rose, Dr. Bach said, would help to bring encouragement to those who felt that life had started to pass them by. Wild Rose people are generally happy as they are, are resistant to change, and, as a result, may pass up chances.

Olive helps to restore strength to those who have suffered great mental or physical trauma. It is one of the most frequently prescribed of all the remedies. So, too, is White Chestnut, which will quiet and eventually put an end to repetitive, distracting thoughts, ideas, and arguments, thus aiding concentration.

If you find yourself suddenly feeling down for no apparent reason, Mustard lifts the gloom that can descend on you quickly, just as if a cold, dark cloud were overshadowing you, and helps to sustain a sense of inner happiness and purpose. Chestnut Bud helps you learn the lessons of daily life more easily and take full advantage of what Dr. Bach defined as "observation and experience."

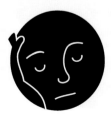

Dreaminess
Clematis people are frequently daydreamers, happier in a world of their own rather than getting the most out of reality.

CLEMATIS

When assessing whether or not you are in a negative Clematis state, the key words that sum up the condition are indifference, dreaminess, lack of attention, and unconsciousness. Clematis people avoid problems and unpleasantness by withdrawing into a world of their own, full of illusions and lacking reality. Such people prefer to be alone with their thoughts, while, whenever they fall ill, they make little or no effort to get well. The state can be sparked off at any time when the mind is occupied with inner problems, worries, and paradoxically, even pleasure. As always, there is a positive aspect to counterbalance the negative. If you are in a positive Clematis state, you will be full of interest in everything that goes on around you, learning from events rather than letting them pass you by.

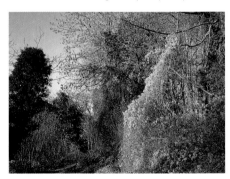

Environment
In the wild, Clematis is frequently found growing in thickets and hedges.

Datafile

BOTANICAL NAME
Clematis vitalba.

HABITAT
Hedges, thickets, and woods, favoring chalky soil and limestone.

PLANT DESCRIPTION
Clematis is a straggly climber. Its fragrant flowers bloom from midsummer to early fall. Strictly speaking, there are no petals as such—instead, there are tonguelike sepals, which are greenish-white in color. They surround a cluster of pale green styles and creamy white stamens.

REMEDY PREPARATION
Sun method.

INDICATIONS FOR USE
Daydreaming; failure to concentrate; escaping from reality; taking little or no interest in the world around you; a lack of vitality; needing a lot of sleep; the tendency to faint.

WHAT TREATMENT SHOULD ACHIEVE
The remedy encourages your artistic and creative tendencies. It also enables you to take an interest in what is going on around you and the important things you can contribute to life as a whole. By making it your mission to join in, rather than stand aloof and self-absorbed, you will gain a better understanding of all the ins and outs of life. You will be master of your thoughts, and start enjoying life and living it to the full.

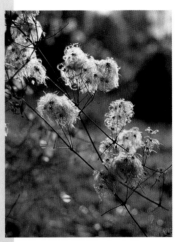

Seeds
The common name for Clematis is "old man's beard," because of its fluffy seed heads.

The Clematis Remedy

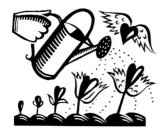

Creativity
*Taking Clematis encourages
the mind's natural fertility.*

Clematis people can seem dreamy and ungrounded. They live with vague thoughts of future happiness, and Dr. Bach once wrote that they spend much of their time dreaming "of ambitions they do not strive to realize." Though "they are generally quiet and gentle…they do not find enough joy in life itself; do not live enough in the present." Nevertheless, on the whole, "they seem contented, being not fully awake, and happy in their dreams of ideals." What it means to be a Clematis type is fairly easy to define in general terms. For one thing, more likely than not you are creative and artistic. You love to have something to anticipate and look forward to— something in the future about which you can hope, dream, and even fantasize. However, the downside of this is that you may lack interest in the here and now, your lack of interest being demonstrated through absentmindedness and inattention. You are also inclined to lack concentration and become easily bored with anything that is not stimulating enough to retain your interest.

Losing touch with reality

If your creative potential cannot be realized, then a negative Clematis state will almost certainly arise. To others, you may well appear to be behaving eccentrically, since you allow yourself to be dominated by illusions that take little or no account of realities. Because you will be attaching little importance to physical things, your health may start to suffer as well. You will nearly always give the impression of being rather sleepy, since Clematis people are really never wholly awake and aware. There is a tendency to take refuge in your dreams, with a consequent loss of contact with reality and what is actually going on in the world around you.

By taking Clematis, you will be able to counter all such negative emotions. The remedy will fill you with the positive energy that you are currently lacking, helping you to gain control of your natural creativity. Your inner drive and sense of purpose will become focused more in the present, while you will put an end to the risk of sinking into a state of semipermanent escapism.

Clematis can also help in cases of fainting. In such circumstances, the best way of administering the remedy is to place a few drops on the lips of the sufferer. It is also an important ingredient of Rescue Remedy (see pages 214–217).

The Negative State

The negative **Clematis** state is characterized by indifference, apathy, dreaminess, and a lack of interest in the present.

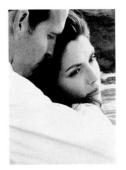

HONEYSUCKLE

If Clematis people tend to daydream about the future, Honeysuckle people, according to Dr. Bach, are the complete opposite. Their tendency is to look to the past, maybe to happier days. As a result, there is the risk of losing interest in the issues and demands of the present, missing out on much of life as a result through a preoccupation with past events and happenings. The remedy will help you by encouraging you to focus more on the present, helping you to put the past into perspective, so that it does not come to dominate your thoughts. Honeysuckle may help bereaved people who think back all the time, or act as if their loved one were still alive.

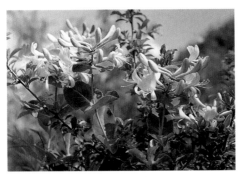

Varieties
There are several Honeysuckle varieties. Dr. Bach used L. caprifolium for his remedy.

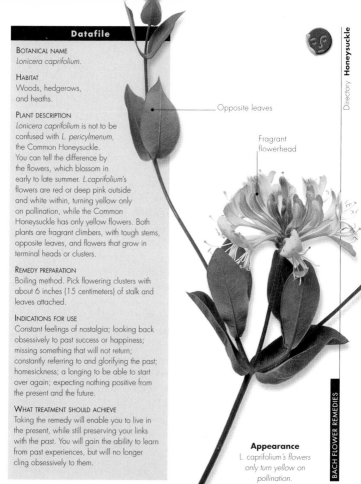

Datafile

BOTANICAL NAME
Lonicera caprifolium.

HABITAT
Woods, hedgerows,
and heaths.

PLANT DESCRIPTION
Lonicera caprifolium is not to be
confused with L. pericylmenum,
the Common Honeysuckle.
You can tell the difference by
the flowers, which blossom in
early to late summer. L.caprifolium's
flowers are red or deep pink outside
and white within, turning yellow only
on pollination, while the Common
Honeysuckle has only yellow flowers. Both
plants are fragrant climbers, with tough stems,
opposite leaves, and flowers that grow in
terminal heads or clusters.

REMEDY PREPARATION
Boiling method. Pick flowering clusters with
about 6 inches (15 centimeters) of stalk and
leaves attached.

INDICATIONS FOR USE
Constant feelings of nostalgia; looking back
obsessively to past success or happiness;
missing something that will not return;
constantly referring to and glorifying the past;
homesickness; a longing to be able to start
over again; expecting nothing positive from
the present and the future.

WHAT TREATMENT SHOULD ACHIEVE
Taking the remedy will enable you to live in
the present, while still preserving your links
with the past. You will gain the ability to learn
from past experiences, but will no longer
cling obsessively to them.

Opposite leaves

Fragrant
flowerhead

Appearance
L. caprifolium's flowers
only turn yellow on
pollination.

The Honeysuckle Remedy

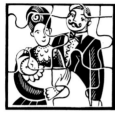

Life's jigsaw
Honeysuckle helps to make sense of the past pieces in life's jigsaw.

Honeysuckle, wrote Dr. Bach, is the remedy "to remove from the mind the regrets and sorrows of the past, to counteract all influences, all wishes and desires of the past, and to bring us back to the present." What this means in practical terms is that the Honeysuckle remedy helps you to avoid becoming obsessively nostalgic. By taking it, although you preserve your links with your past, you no longer cling to them protectively as an insurance policy against the realities of the present and the possibilities of the future. By helping to rebalance your attitudes to past and present, the remedy can ensure

that both are given the chance to hold their appropriate place in your life. The state to avoid is one in which you find yourself living mentally largely in the past, with a consequent lack of ability to step back from it and absorb the lessons it has taught you. These can be an invaluable guide to conduct, both now and in the future.

The lure of the past

The fate of Lot's wife, as described in the Bible, for instance, was a direct consequence of her being a Honeysuckle type. Instead of concentrating her energies on her flight and escape from Sodom, she turned back to face the burning town and was turned into a pillar of salt. Queen Victoria's fanatical devotion to the memory of her husband Prince Albert led her to leave his bedroom at Windsor Castle untouched and to insist on remaining dressed in mourning for the rest of her life—another instance of a Honeysuckle state of mind in action. Such people unconsciously

refuse to see or accept anything new,
a classic giveaway being their
tendency to pepper their conversation
with phrases like "I used to…" and
"When I was still…".

Such a state normally builds up over
a reasonably protracted period,
although it may also be of relatively
short duration, especially where
children are concerned. For instance,
the remedy has often been
recommended to help children at
boarding school get over homesickness.
The state is particularly common in the
elderly, for obvious reasons; here the
remedy helps such people to come to
terms with their current life. Taking the
remedy means that you will be able to
keep your memories alive without losing
sight of the present, at the same time
ensuring that they do not dominate your
thoughts unduly.

The Negative State

The negative **Honeysuckle** state is
characterized by living in the past, with the
refusal to accept anything that is new.

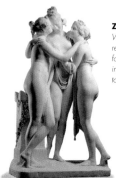

Zest for life
Wild Rose will reawaken your taste for the gracious things in life and encourage you to rise to its challenges.

WILD ROSE
To put it at its bluntest, Wild Rose people have given up the unequal battle. As Dr. Bach himself said, they "have surrendered to the struggle of life without complaint." If you are in a negative Wild Rose state, you will have lost all enthusiasm or ambition to better anything in your life. You are resigned to taking things as they are, without making any effort to change or improve them. What the remedy does is to help to rekindle zest and enthusiasm, reawakening that sleeping sense of vitality. It can benefit people whose lives seem to move along a preset path without anything unexpected ever happening to break the predictability and the consequent boredom.

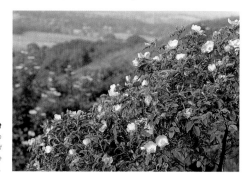

Environment
Wild Rose is also known as the Dog Rose. It grows in thickets on the fringes of woodland.

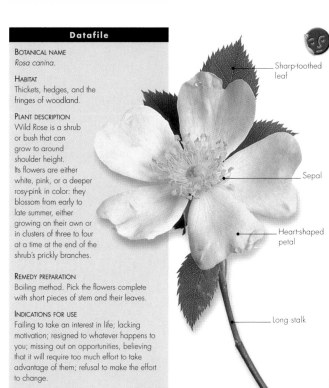

Datafile

BOTANICAL NAME
Rosa canina.

HABITAT
Thickets, hedges, and the fringes of woodland.

PLANT DESCRIPTION
Wild Rose is a shrub or bush that can grow to around shoulder height. Its flowers are either white, pink, or a deeper rosy-pink in color: they blossom from early to late summer, either growing on their own or in clusters of three to four at a time at the end of the shrub's prickly branches.

REMEDY PREPARATION
Boiling method. Pick the flowers complete with short pieces of stem and their leaves.

INDICATIONS FOR USE
Failing to take an interest in life; lacking motivation; resigned to whatever happens to you; missing out on opportunities, believing that it will require too much effort to take advantage of them; refusal to make the effort to change.

WHAT TREATMENT SHOULD ACHIEVE
Taking the remedy helps you to recover the zest for life. It will put an end to feelings of resignation and your willingness to put up with things as they are, both of which are signs of a negative Wild Rose state.

Sharp-toothed leaf

Sepal

Heart-shaped petal

Long stalk

Flowers and fruit
Wild Rose blooms in high summer: it bears fruit in the form of rose hips later in the year.

The Wild Rose Remedy

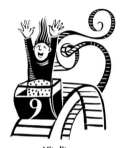

Vitality
Wild Rose helps you to get rid of resignation and start enjoying life.

If you have resigned yourself to illness and its consequences, find the work you do uncongenial, and life in general dull, monotonous, and flat, Wild Rose remedy can help you. Otherwise, you will simply carry on feeling that it is your destiny to put up with whatever is troubling you, rather than taking positive action to alter it. Typically, you are passive, accept life as it is, and take things lying down rather than trying to make a life for yourself.

The power to change things for the better lies in your own hands and taking Wild Rose remedy is the essential first step in unleashing it. Without it, you will just jog along as you are, taking life as it comes, lacking the ambition to change anything—even when, to the outside eye, you are being given an opportunity to change things for the better. Instead, it all seems too much trouble to bother and you prefer to rest on your laurels.

Transforming life

With the remedy's aid, the situation can be completely transformed. Taking it will help you to banish your lack of interest and vitality, and your willingness to accept your lot in life unchallenged, which are prime characteristics of a negative Wild Rose state. Instead, you will find yourself developing a renewed interest in life and in everything that is going on around you.

What the remedy enables you to do, as you will soon notice, is to mobilize your inner reserves and so put back the zest of living into your life. As a consequence of this, you will find yourself enjoying a new sense of inner spiritual and emotional freedom as the barriers come down and you open up your mind to new, varied, and exciting possibilities and opportunities.

You will soon find that as your approach to life starts to become more open and flexible, the benefits will start to accumulate. Now, you are prepared and willing to try out new, positive approaches to getting the most out of all that life has to offer you. Finally, you will begin to realize exactly how to take advantage of all your hitherto latent or suppressed inner potential, and, as you do so, the transformation will become complete.

As with the other Bach remedies, if the condition is associated with other emotional states, then it may be appropriate to take additional measures to treat the complaint.

The Negative State

The negative **Wild Rose** state is characterized by a lack of interest in the direction in which your life is going.

Mental strain
*Olive helps you to cope
with the extremes of mental
exhaustion when everything in
life becomes simply too much.*

OLIVE
When your reserves of spiritual and emotional energy are exhausted Olive helps to restore them. People in a negative Olive state have suffered so much mentally and physically that they end up drained of all strength. Just getting through daily life is hard work; at times, they are scarcely able to keep going. The relentless strains from which they suffer make it impossible for them to enjoy even the simplest pleasures. What the remedy does is to help in the unlocking and rebuilding of your energy stores, reviving mind, body, and spirit. Through this, you will find that you regain the ability to take charge again, and to cope well, rather than give up, when you are faced with complete mental exhaustion.

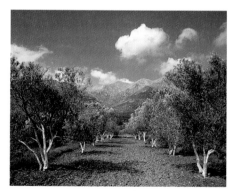

Environment
*Olive does not
grow wild in the US.
The remedy is made in
the Mediterranean.*

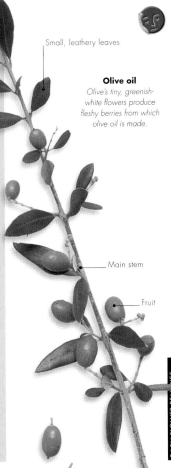

Datafile

BOTANICAL NAME
Olea europaea.

HABITAT
Mediterranean Europe.

PLANT DESCRIPTION
This small evergreen, with characteristic pale gray bark, has tiny, inconspicuous white-green flowers, which bloom in spring. They are carried in clusters, or racemes, with 20 to 30 flowers to each inflorescence.

REMEDY PREPARATION
Sun method.

INDICATIONS FOR USE
Complete mental and physical exhaustion; feeling washed out, and finding everything too much of an effort; deep inner tiredness; needing a lot of sleep; inability to cope with or enjoy everyday life and pleasures because of tiredness.

WHAT TREATMENT SHOULD ACHIEVE
Taking the remedy will enable you to mobilize and restore your inner strength and vitality. Because you will be able to rely on your inner voices to guide you, you will find that you are able to cope even with extreme pressures and demands.

Small, leathery leaves

Olive oil
Olive's tiny, greenish-white flowers produce fleshy berries from which olive oil is made.

Main stem

Fruit

The Olive Remedy

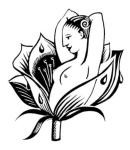

Restorative
*Olive recharges the batteries
when you are exhausted.*

Throughout human history, the olive tree has been a symbol of peace and harmony. In the Bible, for instance, the dove brought an olive branch back to Noah as a sign that the flood had abated and that, as God had promised, evil had been purged and calm and order had returned to the Earth.

The remedy that Dr. Bach prepared from the olive's flowers is one of the most frequently used of all the 38 flower remedies. Its use is called for when it comes to restoring much-needed tranquility to a tired, troubled mind and to rebuilding strength in an exhausted body. Bach practitioners recommend taking olive to help you recover after an illness, especially if you are weak, tired and generally debilitated. The remedy can also help you if you find that your life is so full and demanding that you have little or no time left over for rest and relaxation. If this is your situation, the chances are that you will become increasingly tired, until it reaches the point when there are no reserves of strength or energy left for you to draw on. If you habitually find yourself in this state, what you have to do is to learn how to husband your vital energies, rather than spend them heedlessly. In other words, you need to learn not to overdo things.

Regaining lost energy

If you are in this position, the remedy will help to revive you. Once you have regained your lost energies, you will feel transformed, more than capable of coping with the stresses and strains of life. In fact, to others, it may seem as if you have seemingly inexhaustible energy reserves. This appears to be the case precisely because you have learned how to listen to what your inner feelings are telling you. You have also learned that it is folly to ignore nature's warning signs when they occur.

A key to health

By recognizing and doing something about the needs of your mind and body, you are well on the way to finding the strength you require, as you feel the renewed, revitalized energy flowing into and through you. You will come to appreciate, as Dr. Bach did more than 60 years ago, that health "exists when there is perfect harmony between Soul and mind and body: and that this harmony, and this harmony alone, must be attained before cure can be accomplished."

The Negative State

The negative **Olive** state is characterized by a weak, debilitated, and exhausted body and a tired mind.

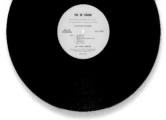

Recurring thoughts
*Because White Chestnut
counters repetitive patterns of
thought, Dr. Bach dubbed it the
"gramophone record remedy."*

WHITE CHESTNUT

If you find that you are suffering mental agonies as a result of worrying, repetitive, and unwanted thoughts, White Chestnut can help you. If you leave things as they are, you will find yourself becoming exhausted and unable to concentrate. In extreme cases, you can become obsessed with worries—even if you do not have a reason to worry, you will find one. There is also an unwillingness to acknowledge the circumstances that led to the development of the overanxiety in the first place. What the remedy does is to help your mind to calm down and regain control. By achieving this, you are able to think positively, and will be far better positioned to find constructive solutions to problems.

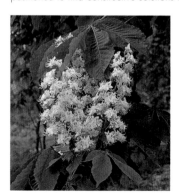

Flowers
*White Chestnut flowers
in dense spikes. The upper
flowers are normally male,
the lower ones female.*

Datafile

BOTANICAL NAME
Aesculus hippocastanum.

HABITAT
Woodland.

PLANT DESCRIPTION
White Chestnut is made from the Horse Chestnut tree's flowers, which are creamy white dappled with crimson and yellow. The flowers grow in dense spikes, which, because the lower flowers have longer stalks than the upper ones, look like pyramids when the tree is in full blossom. The male flowers tend to grow at the top of the spikes, the female ones lower down. The tree blossoms in late spring and early summer.

REMEDY PREPARATION
Sun method. Gather both male and female flowers.

INDICATIONS FOR USE
Persistent worrying thoughts; mental arguments that seem unresolvable; constant preoccupation with problems and their causes; thoughts that recur time and again even though you are doing your conscious best to exclude them from your mind.

WHAT TREATMENT SHOULD ACHIEVE
Taking the remedy will help you to calm down and take an objective view of things going on in your mind. It will stop you being distracted by your thoughts, restore your ability to concentrate, and enable you to enjoy renewed peace of mind. You will also be able to use your powers of thought constructively.

Leaves
By the time they reach maturity, White Chestnut leaves are large and fan-shaped.

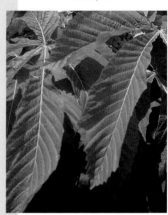

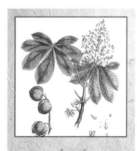

Aesculus Hippocastanum

The White Chestnut Remedy

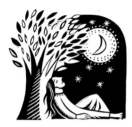

Inner peace
*The remedy frees
the mind from persistent
worrying thoughts.*

White Chestnut people are exceptionally unfortunate. Rather than being victims of others, which is bad enough in itself, they are at the mercy of their own thoughts. Instead of being able to think things through rationally and logically, they are plagued by what seems like a constant, repetitive dialog or even an argument within the mind, as various contradictory ideas and opinions flow backward and forward, seemingly with no chance of any clear-cut resolution.

In fact, things can reach such a pitch that it appears as if the mind has a life of its own, independent of anything going on in the world around it— sufferers often fail to hear what is being said to them, even if they are being addressed directly.

Signs and symptoms

If you recognize these psychological signs, it is likely that you will be familiar with the physical ones as well. You may have problems getting to sleep at night or your thoughts may wake you up again in the early hours of the morning, refusing to leave you alone and go away. Mental overactivity can lead to depression and fatigue, associated with a lack of concentration.

By taking White Chestnut, you are taking the first steps toward calming things down, getting your brain back to normal and reestablishing logical, clear patterns of thought within it. You can then start tidying your overcluttered mind, sorting out the important from the unimportant, and establishing some basic priorities in your thought processes. It is like clearing out a cupboard—you will be surprised just how much you can do without once you have put your mind to it.

After you have done this successfully, you will no longer be a prisoner of your thoughts, but will be back in control of them once again. Eventually, you will reach the stage where you are at peace with yourself and the world around you. Not only will you have learned how to remain in charge and harness your powers of imagination— you will have discovered how to put them to positive use. What is more, you will have recovered your former mental and physical energy.

The Negative State

The negative **White Chestnut** state is characterized by mental overactivity and unstoppable thoughts.

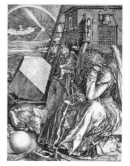

Depression
Mustard helps to deal with depressions that suddenly arise, lift, and then, some time later, strike you down again.

MUSTARD
If you suffer from the kind of depression that comes on you suddenly, descending like a dark cloud hiding all the sunshine that brings joy to life, then Mustard is the remedy for you. If the mood persists, you sink into a state of complete misery, especially since you cannot identify any reason for your deep unhappiness. The first thing to understand about Mustard depression is that it has no cause. More than this, it can come and go almost as it likes, lasting for days, weeks, and even months at a time. Then, it lifts as quickly as it came, only to recur again in an unpredictable cycle. What the remedy does is to dispel all the negative clouds by reinforcing the inner senses of joy and purposefulness. As Dr. Bach put it, "this remedy dispels gloom, and brings joy into life."

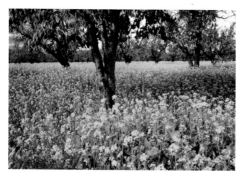

Treatment
Dr. Bach used Wild Mustard, or Charlock, to treat sudden depression.

Datafile

BOTANICAL NAME
Sinapsis arvensis.

HABITAT
Fields and along roads.

PLANT DESCRIPTION
Wild Mustard is an annual, clearly identifiable by its brilliant yellow flowers, which appear from late spring to midsummer. The flowers start off as short spikes, which soon develop into long, beaded pods. The stems of the plant are often covered with rough, short hairs.

REMEDY PREPARATION
Boiling method. Pick the flower-heads above the faded blooms and seed pods.

INDICATIONS FOR USE
Feelings of intense sadness, melancholy, depression, and misery that strike and then go for no apparent reason.

WHAT TREATMENT SHOULD ACHIEVE
Long-term stability, ongoing happiness and tranquility, and an inner calm that seems unshakeable and certainly cannot be shattered or destroyed easily. People who have taken the remedy will tell you that the feeling it promotes is like that of slowly waking from a dark, heavy dream and taking the first steps into the light.

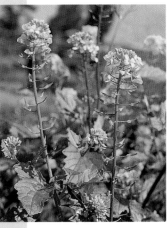

Harvesting
You need to pick the flowers before the seed pods start forming. This happens soon after the plant blooms.

The Mustard Remedy

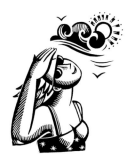

Light and joy
The Mustard remedy will lift the clouds of sudden, acute depression.

If you suffer from depression, dark moods, and dejection—all of which strike without any warning or apparent cause—then you are in a negative Mustard state and you need to take urgent steps to relieve it. The phenomenon is not only deeply upsetting for you personally, but it can also affect your family and friends, who themselves may well get depressed by the extent of your sufferings, which can be extreme. Sufferers from Mustard depression can be driven right to the

brink of total despair, unable to think of anything that can help to cheer them up, or relieve the mood. Nothing seems worthwhile—on the contrary, everything seems hopeless and simply not worth bothering about.

The extremes of despair

If you are experiencing a full-blown attack of Mustard depression, life is unutterably awful for you. It is almost impossible to put a brave face on things and wear a false mask of happiness or cheerfulness, covering things up as you might find it possible to do in a negative Agrimony state.

What Winston Churchill, himself a sufferer from this kind of depression, eloquently termed the "black dog" of despair has taken over, cutting you off from the rest of the world, and effectively taking all the light and joy out of your life. You are very much on your own, alone with your sufferings.

Even more frustratingly, as Dr. Bach himself noted, "it may not be possible to give any reason or explanation of such attacks." Just as much to the point, unlike the doubt and discouragement that characterize a negative Gentian state or the hopelessness that is typical of the Gorse one, the Mustard state of mind can strike out of the blue—even when the facts tell you that, logically, you should be feeling happy, satisfied and secure. Nor is there any immediate light at the end of the tunnel. Although the depression may lift just as suddenly as it came, it is so severe while it lasts that nothing else in life seems to matter; all your thoughts turn in on yourself.

The Mustard remedy starts by helping to dispel the clouds of gloom that are overwhelming and suffocating you, so lifting the effects of the melancholia or depression that are both characteristic of the negative Mustard state. Longer term, it will help you to develop inner stability and tranquility.

The Negative State

The negative **Mustard** state is characterized by depression that seems to have no real reason behind it.

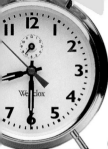

Repeating mistakes

The alarm goes and you're late again. Chestnut Bud is the remedy you need if you are to overcome the inability to learn from experience.

CHESTNUT BUD

If you are one of those people who seemed fated never to learn from experience—either your own or that of others—the Chestnut Bud remedy can help you. As Dr. Bach wrote, this remedy "is to help us to take full advantage of our daily experiences, and to see ourselves, and our mistakes, as others do." With its aid, you will be able to overcome your seeming inability to learn from your experiences and mistakes, or from others'. Instead, you will find yourself able to recognize and benefit from all that life has to teach you, growing and developing in character as a result. The alternative is to continue to hold back, approaching life principally on a trial-and-error basis, so failing to profit from all that you could have learned in the future.

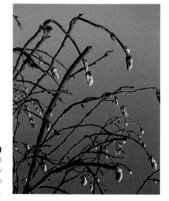

Budding

In early spring, the buds gradually swell until they are ready for picking in mid- to late spring.

Datafile

BOTANICAL NAME
Aesculus hippocastanum.

HABITAT
Woodland.

PLANT DESCRIPTION
The Horse Chestnut tree, from which the White Chestnut remedy comes, is also the source of the Chestnut Bud remedy. In this instance, you need to look for the tree's large, sticky, glossy buds in around mid- to late spring. They are ready to harvest once they have begun to swell. The sign of this starting is when the folded leaves at the top become covered with down, which is discarded as the leaves expand.

REMEDY PREPARATION
Boiling method. Pick the bud and about 6 inches (15 centimeters) of twig.

INDICATIONS FOR USE
Slowness to learn even from repeated experiences; making the same mistakes over and over again; not getting enough out of experiences; failing to benefit from the experience of others; not learning the lessons of the past.

WHAT TREATMENT SHOULD ACHIEVE
Taking the remedy should give you the ability to analyze and learn from events, actions, and behavior of the past. It will also help you to step back and assess things from a different perspective and to view your own experiences and those of others impartially.

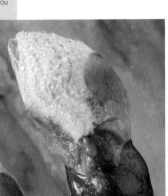

Harvesting
When the leaves throw off their down, the buds can be harvested for the Chestnut Bud remedy.

The Chestnut Bud Remedy

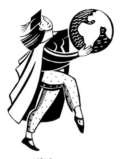

Life lessons
*Chestnut Bud helps you
to learn from experience
and the lessons of life.*

Made from the same tree as White Chestnut, the Chestnut Bud remedy, as its name implies, is derived from the Horse Chestnut tree's sticky buds. These are harvested in midspring at the time when they are just starting to open. The remedy will help you if, like many people, you find it hard to learn from experience. You may, for instance, continue to buy clothes that you know, in your heart of hearts, are basically unsuited to you, so each new outfit takes its place in turn with its almost identical fellows in your closet, never to see the light of day again. Things like this are not going to stop unless you come round to accepting the view that, after all, there is something useful to learn from the past. Instead, you will simply go on and on as you have been doing, even though the end result will almost always be the same. What this means is that, whatever your experiences, it seems as if they are not being digested properly and not enough is being learned from them as a result. Nor does it ever seem to occur to you that it is worthwhile trying to learn from the experiences of others.

Looking for insight

Some of this may be down to an unconscious lack of insight, which means that it may be easier for a candid friend to spot your need for the remedy than it is for you to realize that it can help you. To help yourself, you should make the resolution to try to learn something new from every experience. One way of doing this is to set aside time at the end of the day to review what has happened to you and ascertain what you can learn from it.

The remedy gives you the ability to appreciate the consequences of your actions more clearly, so that you can use them as a basis for positive growth. In fact, by developing the ability to watch and learn—particularly from others—you will gain in knowledge, wisdom, and insight, making it easier to avoid errors of judgment in the first place. Slowly, but surely, you will find your mental flexibility increasing as you become a good learner. This is particularly important, because it helps us to move forward spiritually and emotionally. Chestnut Bud can be a vital remedy when our progress is stalled, helping us to grow and evolve and so get the most out of our lives.

The Negative State

The negative **Chestnut Bud** state is characterized by an inability to learn from experience by repeating mistakes often.

REMEDIES IN ACTION

By this point, you will have come to realize for yourself not only how beautifully simple the Bach system of healing is, but how easy it is to master its principles and to put them into practice successfully. What, at all times, you should remember first and foremost is Dr. Bach's belief that "the mind is the most sensitive part of our bodies, and hence the best guide to tell us what remedy is required." By now, you should also be starting to appreciate just how the 38 remedies Dr. Bach discovered in his great quest through the fields, forests, and hillsides combine and interact to deal with practically every possible condition.

Case Study

Alison felt very uncomfortable about her appearance, and was constantly dieting, relapsing, and regaining all the weight she had taken off. Since her mother's death she had also become extremely restless, vulnerable and unable to rest and relax.

Impatiens was advised to ease Alison's restlessness and general impatience, together with **Vervain**, **Crab Apple**, **Rock Water**, **Clematis**, **Honeysuckle**, and **Star of Bethlehem** (the last for the shock of losing her mother). Later, **White Chestnut** and **Beech** were added and the **Honeysuckle** and **Star of Bethlehem** discontinued.

As the situation altered and improved, the mixture changed accordingly, with the addition of **Scleranthus**, to help her with her fluctuating moods. She was soon feeling better and eating more sensibly and was developing more balanced eating patterns.

Case Study

Nick was suffering from a complete lack of mental and physical energy—so much so that daily life had come to a standstill. The problem had started a year back and had gradually become worse.

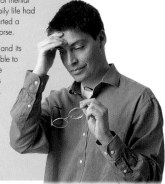

Olive was the obvious remedy of choice and its effects were immediate. It was then possible to probe into Nick's state of mind further. He had suffered many disappointments in his business life, which made him feel angry, let down, and despondent. The practitioner he had consulted added **Walnut**, **Vervain**, **White Chestnut**, **Willow**, **Star of Bethlehem**, and **Vine** to the list. Eventually, as matters improved, this was cut back to **Vine**, **Walnut**, **Olive**, and **Willow**.

Case Study

Bianca suffered from acute depression mainly because she felt unattractive and seemed to be incapable of sustaining any relationship. She became upset easily, especially as her boyfriend had just left her.

Star of Bethlehem was chosen to help Bianca cope with the shock she was feeling at the loss of her boyfriend, plus **Chestnut Bud**, since it was not the first time this had happened. **Elm** was advised to help restore her natural confidence, **Gentian** to deal with the discouragement she was feeling, and **Red Chestnut** to help put her feelings for others into perspective.

Later the remedy mixture was revised, with **Star of Bethlehem**, **Elm**, and **Gentian** being discontinued, and **Centaury**, **Willow**, and **Larch** substituted. Gradually, she began to take positive steps to overcome her problems.

Remedies for Loneliness

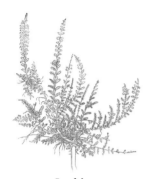

Fearful
*Heather helps to deal with
the loneliness that you mask
with companionship.*

Dr. Bach identified and incorporated three distinct definitions of loneliness into his system of healing. There are quite marked differences between them.

Water Violet people, for example, are quite happy to be solitary types because they possess great inner reserves of peace and serenity. These enable them to be self-reliant—they are perfectly prepared to carry on down their own paths alone. Certainly, they would never dream of bothering others

with their problems. They are quiet and capable, but reserved. The downside is that they often feel themselves to be superior to others, sometimes coming across as being proud and aloof.

Impatiens people also tend to be loners, keeping others at a distance, so that they can get on with whatever it is that they have to do faster, without outside interference. As Dr. Bach put it, they "often prefer to think and work alone, so that they can do everything at their own speed" and in their own way. Although intelligent, capable, and quick-witted, Impatiens people can come across as being impatient and irritable with others, since they fail to appreciate that outsiders can make equally valuable contributions to what is in hand. Even though they may be slower in their approach, they may well be more methodical than Impatiens types.

Seeking companionship

Heather people, in contrast, are the complete opposite. Dr. Bach described them as "always seeking the companionship of anyone who may be available, as they find it necessary to discuss their own affairs with others, no matter whom it may be. They are very unhappy if they have to be alone for any length of time."

Heather people are suffering from an overwhelming fear of being alone, and if allowed, they are liable to start telling you their entire life story as soon as they meet you. In fact, the state can be an extremely selfish one. People in a negative Heather state will happily chatter away about themselves for hour after hour—it was not for nothing that Dr. Bach nicknamed them "buttonholers" —but they seem to be incapable of listening to and learning from anything others might have to say to them.

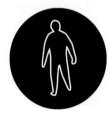

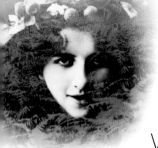

Aloof and reserved

*Water Violet will help if you
have withdrawn into yourself,
preferring to be on your own
rather than with others.*

WATER VIOLET

If you are quiet, aloof, and reserved, with a tendency to withdraw into yourself, especially if you frequently prefer spending time away from the company of others and on your own, you are a classic Water Violet person. You are extremely independent, tending to immerse yourself in your own activities, and enjoying the freedom to follow your preferred pursuits. Sometimes, though, you can appear proud and others might think you to be somewhat snobbish. What the Water Violet remedy does is to help boost your inner sensitivities so that you become more aware of others and prepared to share experiences with them.

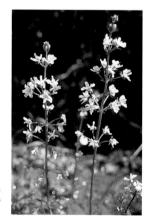

Harvesting

*Water Violet can be
difficult to gather since it
often grows in midstream.*

Datafile

BOTANICAL NAME
Hottonia palustris.

HABITAT
Slow-moving or stagnant streams,
pools, and ditches.

PLANT DESCRIPTION
Water Violet actually grows in water,
which can make it problematic to gather.
Its small, delicate flowers blossom from
late spring to early summer, depending
on the weather. They grow in whorls one
above the other around a leafless stalk.
Though the plant does have leaves,
these remain invisible below the
water's surface.

REMEDY PREPARATION
Sun method.

INDICATIONS FOR USE
Wanting at times to withdraw completely
from life in order to be on your own to
enjoy your own company; feeling
yourself to be superior to others, but at
the same time isolated and lonely,
because people have taken your reserve as
a sign that you are conceited or supercilious.

WHAT TREATMENT SHOULD ACHIEVE
The remedy will help you to feel comfortable
with yourself, sure in the knowledge that you
generally have life well in hand. It will also
encourage you to develop a more open attitude
toward others, so that they see you as a well
balanced and independent-minded individual.
You will be seen as a wise counselor, who is
able to create a positive atmosphere charged
with calm, confidence, and tranquility.

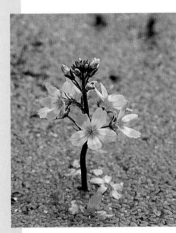

Flowers
*Water Violet flowers are
unmistakable, with their
prominent central eyes
around which the petals
are arranged.*

The Water Violet Remedy

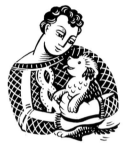

Isolation
*Water Violet helps
break down barriers
and end isolation.*

According to Dr. Bach, the positive qualities of Water Violet people far outweigh the negative ones. Such people, he wrote, are "often clever and talented. Their peace and calmness is a blessing to those around them." Putting all their many capabilities at the service of others, they are "tranquil, sympathetic, wise, practical counselors, who have poise and dignity and pass gracefully through life." Like the Water Violet plant itself, Water Violet people stand proud, tall, and on their own. They tend to keep themselves to themselves, so, although they are willing to give advice if asked, they do not try to interfere with or influence others. The balance between positive and negative within them, however, can sometimes be tenuous, and this is especially evident in their relationships.

Inside your shell

If you are in a negative Water Violet state, it is all too easy for you to withdraw into yourself, shutting yourself off from others in a form of self-imposed isolation, though it may be that you simply prefer your own company.

When you are like this, however, others may see you in a negative light. They may assume, for instance, that you are being stand-offish, remote, and unapproachable, because you make it very hard for others to break through the barriers you have set up around yourself. This means that they find it difficult to establish any contact point, however tenuous, with you, on which it might be possible to build at least the semblance of some form of relationship. In the words of Greta Garbo, you "want to be alone."

As far as you are concerned, despite your undoubted self-sufficiency, you may well start to feel isolated and lonely should the state persist. You may also find yourself becoming more rigid mentally. In such circumstances, the remedy will help you by breaking down negative Water Violet traits and allowing the positive ones to reassert themselves. By enabling you to break down barriers, it will help you to relate better to others and nurture your new-found openness. Rather than deliberately keeping yourself at a distance, you will dispel any negative feelings toward you and develop the ability to inspire them with your poise, wisdom, and quiet confidence.

The Negative State

The negative **Water Violet** state is characterized by a withdrawal from others and self-imposed isolation and aloofness.

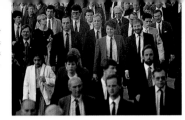

Irritability
Getting irritated by others is a clear sign that Impatiens may be needed.

IMPATIENS

As a mood remedy, Impatiens has many applications. Dr. Bach advised its use "at all times where there is impatience." He stated that "the restfulness this brings hastens recovery"—indeed, he chose it as an ingredient for Rescue Remedy precisely because of its calming effects. Impatiens is also called for if your ability to think on your feet makes everyone else seem dull and slow to you. Nervous frustration will make your inner tensions rise and you will find it harder and harder to give things enough time to take their course. You will find yourself prone to anger, and your moods will make you curt and brusque with others. By reinforcing your hidden reserves of patience and understanding, the remedy will help you to slow down and regain your inner poise.

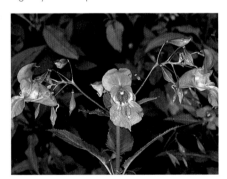

Color
Impatiens varies in color from pale mauve through to a reddish-crimson. You will find this plant along river-banks.

126

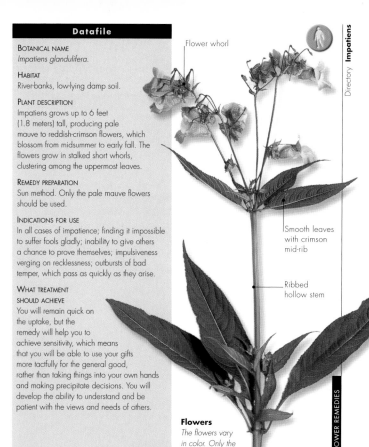

Datafile

BOTANICAL NAME
Impatiens glandulifera.

HABITAT
River-banks, low-lying damp soil.

PLANT DESCRIPTION
Impatiens grows up to 6 feet
(1.8 meters) tall, producing pale
mauve to reddish-crimson flowers, which
blossom from midsummer to early fall. The
flowers grow in stalked short whorls,
clustering among the uppermost leaves.

REMEDY PREPARATION
Sun method. Only the pale mauve flowers
should be used.

INDICATIONS FOR USE
In all cases of impatience; finding it impossible
to suffer fools gladly; inability to give others
a chance to prove themselves; impulsiveness
verging on recklessness; outbursts of bad
temper, which pass as quickly as they arise.

**WHAT TREATMENT
SHOULD ACHIEVE**
You will remain quick on
the uptake, but the
remedy will help you to
achieve sensitivity, which means
that you will be able to use your gifts
more tactfully for the general good,
rather than taking things into your own hands
and making precipitate decisions. You will
develop the ability to understand and be
patient with the views and needs of others.

Flower whorl

Smooth leaves
with crimson
mid-rib

Ribbed
hollow stem

Flowers
*The flowers vary
in color. Only the
palest ones should
be used for the
remedy.*

The Impatiens Remedy

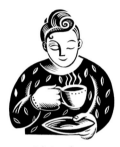

Calming down
Impatiens helps counter irritability and the impatience sparking it.

Are you a workaholic who likes to work alone because, in your view, this is the best way of getting things done faster? If this description fits you, there is the danger that you may be in a negative Impatiens state and need to consider taking a course of Impatiens remedy urgently. This will help you to counter your inability to delegate and your preference to do everything for yourself. You also may be obsessed with work to the exclusion of practically everything else, and impatient and distrustful of others. As a result, you are lonely—the kind of loneliness that comes from being alone at the top, or the loneliness of the long-distance runner, racing far ahead of the field in an attempt to beat the record for the marathon.

Recognizing the state

Someone in a negative Impatiens state is usually fairly easy to spot, for such people are naturally extrovert and demonstrative. If they do not reveal themselves verbally, they will frequently do so through their body language—the nervous drumming of fingers on a tabletop, for instance, or constantly looking at their watch, particularly when someone else is talking to them, are classic negative Impatiens traits.

In general, Impatiens people are quick to think and quick to act. They are also extremely independent. Sometimes, they run the risk of pushing themselves to extremes. If this happens, they can exhaust themselves mentally and physically if they do not make the time to take a step back, rest, and relax. The remedy is a great calmer, which is the reason why Dr. Bach included it in Rescue Remedy (see pages 214–217). For all these reasons, taking Impatiens as a mood remedy is advisable whenever you feel yourself falling into the state even on a short-term basis. Taking it if you are an Impatiens type and in a negative Impatiens state is even more advisable. Either way, the remedy helps you by making you much more patient and tolerant, especially when it comes to dealing with others. Otherwise, you may well end up hurting their feelings. It will enable you to slow down, rather than expect everything to happen instantly.

It will also encourage you to think with your heart as well as your head. With its aid, you will be able to find out just how enjoyable life can be when you take things at a more normal rate.

The Negative State

The negative **Impatiens** state is characterized by a desire to get things done quickly.

HEATHER

If you have ever been button-holed by someone who persists in talking about himself or herself and does not seem to be listening to a word you say in reply, then you have met someone in a typically negative Heather state. Heather people are always on the look-out for an audience: they crave attention since they actively fear being on their own. Unfortunately, their self-obsessive persistence serves only to drive people away from them, thus leading to the isolation and loneliness that they are most frightened of. Taking the Heather remedy helps by putting things in perspective, so problems can be seen for what they are. Those in the positive Heather state become more open to others and less focused on themselves as a result.

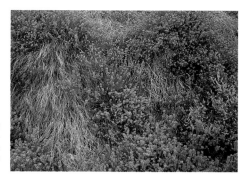

Blossoms

Scotch Heather blossoms from midsummer to early fall.

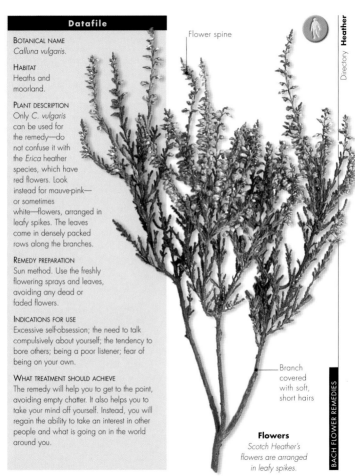

Datafile

BOTANICAL NAME
Calluna vulgaris.

HABITAT
Heaths and
moorland.

PLANT DESCRIPTION
Only *C. vulgaris*
can be used for
the remedy—do
not confuse it with
the *Erica* heather
species, which have
red flowers. Look
instead for mauve-pink—
or sometimes
white—flowers, arranged in
leafy spikes. The leaves
come in densely packed
rows along the branches.

REMEDY PREPARATION
Sun method. Use the freshly
flowering sprays and leaves,
avoiding any dead or
faded flowers.

INDICATIONS FOR USE
Excessive self-obsession; the need to talk
compulsively about yourself; the tendency to
bore others; being a poor listener; fear of
being on your own.

WHAT TREATMENT SHOULD ACHIEVE
The remedy will help you to get to the point,
avoiding empty chatter. It also helps you to
take your mind off yourself. Instead, you will
regain the ability to take an interest in other
people and what is going on in the world
around you.

Flower spine

Branch
covered
with soft,
short hairs

Flowers
Scotch Heather's
flowers are arranged
in leafy spikes.

The Heather Remedy

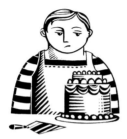

Loneliness
Heather people tend to be self-obsessed and lonely as a result.

Heather people run the risk of becoming obsessive. In the negative Heather state, they are concerned solely with themselves and their own personal problems. They can talk about these for literally hours at a time, almost without pausing for breath.

In extreme cases, even complete strangers can be drawn in—Heather people may well give in to the irresistible urge to offload all their problems onto others. Doing this, however, can be extremely counter-productive in establishing and maintaining any kind of relationship with other people. Heather people frequently find themselves being avoided once the word has got around that they are complete bores. This, however, only aggravates the underlying fear of being on their own, which is also one of their chief worries.

Learning to give, not take

Put at its most basic, Heather people need to develop the ability to give as well as to take. Once you have regained a positive Heather state, you will find yourself just as good a listener as you were a talker. You will develop a sense of empathy with others, finding yourself able to take their concerns just as seriously as you do your own.

You will also develop a greater sense of security, which, in turn, will enable you to create an atmosphere with which others can feel at ease, rather than one that puts them off even approaching you. You also will find that you can put your past experiences to good use, since now you will understand exactly why it is so important to be prepared to listen to and help others. This new-found unselfishness will help to win you many new friends, and win back the ones that might have started to avoid you.

As well as being the type remedy that should be used to deal with the kind of situation described above, Heather is also often recommended as a mood remedy. There are times when everyone suffers from a Heather state of mind. In such circumstances, problems and difficulties can get blown out of all proportion, sometimes to the point when they may seem completely out of control and we simply have to tell someone about it.

In such cases, the Heather remedy acts quickly to get things back to normal. It will help you recognize selfish concerns for what they are, and put an end to them.

The Negative State

The negative **Heather** state is characterized by talkative people with a sole concern for themselves and their own problems.

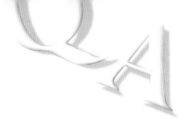

QUESTIONS & ANSWERS

A significant attribute of the Bach remedies is that, as Dr. Bach wrote in *The Twelve Healers and Four Helpers*, "being herbs of Nature they treat our natures … it is because there is something wrong in our natures that disease is able to attack us, and it is this something wrong which the herbs put right, and thus not only heal our bodies, but make us happier and healthier in every way." Many orthodox doctors still find this a difficult notion to comprehend, arguing that, if the remedies work at all, they simply have a placebo effect. This is one of the issues dealt with here.

Q When I told my doctor I was taking Bach remedies, she dismissed them completely, saying "We don't know what they put in these drugs", and "anyway they are only placebos at best." Can you help me by setting my mind at rest? Are they safe to take?

A *First of all, experience shows that the remedies are perfectly safe. They have been used successfully for more than 60 years without any ill effects and to the benefit of patients. Chemical analysis of the bottles shows that there is only brandy and water in them (the active ingredient is the life remedy of the plant,*

which does not show up using standard chemical tests). Nor is there any mystery as to what goes into each remedy—it is made from the plant that is listed on the label, with the addition of the alcohol as part of the brandy, water—and nothing else. They definitely cannot be classified as drugs.

Q I am flying long-haul to Australia shortly. Will any of the remedies prevent jet lag, or help me cope with its symptoms?

A *Taking Walnut may help in adjusting to the changes, with Olive for the tiredness. You could add other remedies depending on your feelings, before and after the flight; Mimulus will help if you are afraid of flying, for example.*

Q Are there any successful examples of treating allergies—or the possible spiritual conditions that may be causing them—with the Bach remedies?

A *Basically, you approach allergies as you would any other condition: you look at the individual involved and his or her state of mind, rather than the physical problem.*

Q Can Bach remedies help with weight loss?

A *No, there is no particular remedy that could be used to reduce weight. A Bach practitioner would treat the emotions that accompany weight problems. Crab Apple supports someone suffering from poor self-image, Gentian would help someone dissatisfied with the results of a diet, and Impatiens would give a dieter patience.*

Q Could you tell me which remedies would benefit someone suffering from anxiety and panic attacks?

A *The two main possibilities are Mimulus and Aspen.*

The former is for known fears, the latter for those of unknown origin. If there seem to be elements of both types of fear involved, try taking both remedies together.

Q If I select three of four remedies, do I mix them together in a single bottle or does each need its own bottle?

A *You can do either—the potency of the remedies is not affected.*

135

Remedies for Oversensitivity

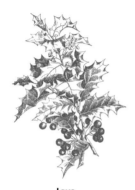

Love

Holly is the remedy of love,
an effective counter to hatred.

What Dr. Bach meant by "oversensitivity" was, as he said, the tendency to be hypersensitive to "influences and ideas." He discovered four separate remedies to deal with the varying aspects of the problem: Agrimony, Holly, Centaury, and Walnut. Agrimony is suggested if you are enduring intense emotional suffering, but putting a brave face on it.

Hatred and its counter

If, on the other hand, you are suffering from negative feelings and thoughts about other people that are so acute that they start to manifest themselves in explosive outbursts of anger, jealousy, hatred, suspicion, and a desire for revenge, then the Holly remedy will help you to deal with the situation.

Being aware of why you are taking such an remedy actually aids in the work of healing. Understanding it will help you to understand more about yourself and what are your inner strengths and weaknesses. This, in turn, helps you to position yourself ready for positive change. By studying the description of each remedy carefully, you will soon be able to decide which remedy—or remedies—are appropriate for you. This applies especially if, as with Holly, there is the potential for confusion, since the term "anger" without qualification can be applied to states of mind other than the specific one described here.

Submissive states

Centaury will help you if you find it difficult, or even impossible, to stand up for yourself, always giving way to others instead. It is a state of submissiveness and docility, which, if carried to extremes, can lead to losing your sense of identity.

Walnut will help to put you back on track if you are susceptible to outside influences. It also makes coming to terms with change and its various consequences easier. It can help if, for instance, you are changing jobs or facing a major milestone in life, such as pregnancy and childbirth, or the time of life leading up to menopause.

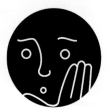

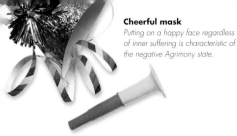

AGRIMONY

People who hide their inner feelings behind a mask of cheerfulness are in the negative Agrimony state. Outsiders rarely discover the worries and anxieties that lie deep within. As Dr. Bach put it, "they hide their cares behind their humor and jesting and are considered very good friends to know." The remedy helps people in this state to consider things more objectively, and to communicate more freely with others.

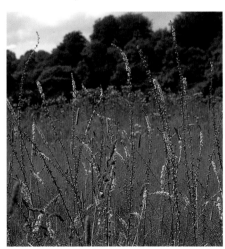

Environment
Agrimony is common in the wild, particularly on wasteland.

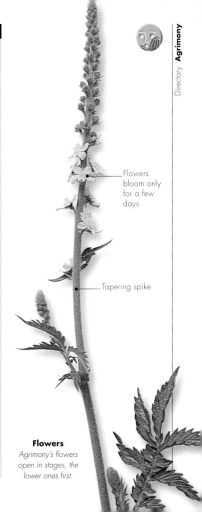

BOTANICAL NAME
Agrimonia eupatoria.

HABITAT
Fields, hedgerows, and wasteland.

PLANT DESCRIPTION
Agrimony's tiny yellow flowers blossom
between June and August. Each flower, which
is attached to a tapering spike by a short stalk
of its own, blooms for only a short time.
The lower buds open first, followed by the
upper ones. The plant has toothed, oval
leaves which produce a yellow dye.

REMEDY PREPARATION
Sun method. Pick the flowering spike and
end buds above any dead or faded flowers.

INDICATIONS FOR USE
Concealing worries behind a facade of
cheerfulness; inability to share difficulties,
anxieties, and problems; avoiding being
alone and instead taking refuge in social
activity; playing down discomfort when ill.

WHAT TREATMENT SHOULD ACHIEVE
Agrimony helps you to relax within yourself,
improving your ability to deal with your
problems more effectively. It is your key to
finding inner calm and peace, so that you
can view the world with genuine good
humor and peace of mind.

Flowers
bloom only
for a few
days

Tapering spike

Flowers
*Agrimony's flowers
open in stages, the
lower ones first.*

The Agrimony Remedy

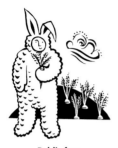

Public face
Agrimony gaiety only serves to cloak deep inner sufferings.

People in need of Agrimony have two faces—one public and the other private. Inwardly, they are troubled and tormented by anxieties and fears, which they try to conceal not only from others but also sometimes even from themselves. Often, these are material worries about things such as illness, financial problems, and difficulties at work. Outwardly, they put a brave face on things to the world.

In a negative Agrimony state, although you appear carefree and untroubled on the surface, underneath you are finding it increasingly difficult to cope and are secretly suffering emotionally and spiritually as a result. Rather than facing up to this, however, you are inclined to cover things up.

Surface appearances

The more difficult things become, the more likely it is that you will make increasing efforts to keep up outward appearances. In fact, even in the most painful of circumstances, you will still be trying to see the funny side of things.

As a result, you will win yourself the reputation of being the life and soul of the party. You will also be prepared to make sacrifices for the sake of peace and quiet, avoiding the possibility of confrontation with others at all costs.

Keeping the ball in the air

More than this, you always have to be on the move, keeping yourself fully occupied to stop yourself having to sit back and think. The impression you make on others is also really important to you—you will go out of your way to court popularity—while you will be constantly seeking out company to take you out of yourself.

It is more than likely that Agrimony people will fall victim to the temptation of taking their problems too lightly. As a result, they can be reluctant to make any serious effort to resolve them, preferring to battle on instead. Taking the remedy will help by transforming all the negatives that are making life a misery for you into positives.

Rather than suppressing negative experiences, which may serve only to aggravate the suffering, you will be able to come to terms with them as you gain the inner strength and stability to deal with the problems that have been besetting you. Ultimately, you will be able to see life in perspective, preserving your sense of humor but doing away with the need to maintain a false façade.

The Negative State

The negative **Agrimony** state is characterized by underlying troubles that you hide with a smile.

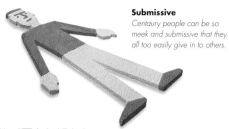

Submissive
Centaury people can be so meek and submissive that they all too easily give in to others.

CENTAURY
Although talented and capable, Centaury people sometimes fail to achieve as much as they could and should. This is because they are submissive, open to being dominated by others, rather than taking charge of their own destiny and initiating things for themselves. The remedy helps them to define their boundaries, so that they know when to give and when to take. It also helps such people to maintain their sense of individuality and to stand up for themselves and their needs.

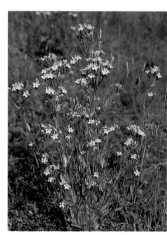

Blossoming
Centaury's flowers come into blossom in tufts.

Datafile

BOTANICAL NAME
Centaurium umbellatum.

HABITAT
Dry fields, roadsides, and wasteland.

PLANT DESCRIPTION
Centaury is an annual, which blooms from early to late summer. Its pink, star-shaped flowers, which grow in clusters, open only on bright, sunny days.

REMEDY PREPARATION
Sun method.

INDICATIONS FOR USE
Lacking the willpower to refuse the demands other people may make on you; being passive, weak-willed, easily exploited, and allowing yourself to be treated as a doormat; lacking the ability to stand up for yourself; and instead suppressing your own wishes and needs.

WHAT TREATMENT SHOULD ACHIEVE
Centaury will help you to assert yourself when you need to and to know when to give in to others and when not to do so. By safeguarding your personality, you will find yourself able to stand up for yourself and your needs. You will come to realize that it is you— and you alone—who is responsible for your progress through life.

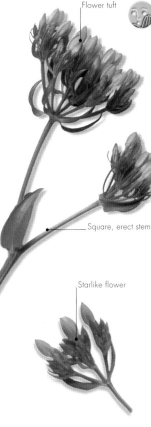

Flower tuft

Square, erect stem

Starlike flower

Flowers
*The flowers open only
when the weather is fine.*

The Centaury Remedy

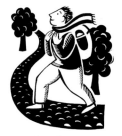

Assertiveness
Centaury helps you to
stride out and overcome
your diffidence.

In *The Twelve Healers and Four Helpers*, Dr. Bach summed up Centaury people as "meek, submissive, and imposed upon because of their good natures." What this means in practice is that, if you are in a negative Centaury state, it may be all too easy for you to fall under the influence of a stronger outside personality, who will take advantage of your innate helpfulness and mildness to exploit you.

The physical consequence of this is that you will often find yourself facing extreme tiredness as a result of overwork, having taken on too much in your desire to be as helpful as possible. Dr. Bach was quick to notice this possibility as well, when he wrote that "even in illness, they may be too willing to help others and get tired and worn-out by their efforts."

What you really want

At the same time, because of your submissiveness and inability to stand up for yourself and your own best interests, you are probably not getting as much as you want out of life. Indeed, you may be on the wrong path altogether, since you find it difficult, or even impossible, to say "No" when the chips are down. The son who allows himself to be persuaded to follow in his father's footsteps and take on the family business, rather than pursuing his own vocation, or the daughter who turns down a marriage proposal, instead sacrificing herself to look after her aging, but dominant, parents, are both classic Centaury types. In this second instance, there is a fine line between

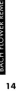

being responsible and being exploited, which, in many instances, is often crossed, or deliberately blurred.

What the remedy does

Inwardly, Centaury people can be mentally alert, active, and fully aware, which only adds to the problems they are having in asserting themselves enough to begin to start leading their own life. While they inwardly know what they should be doing, they lack the strength to start going about it.

It is a matter of priorities. The remedy will give you the strength you need to resolve the dilemma. Taking it will enable you to concentrate on reasserting your individuality. You will also realize that it is, in fact, possible to combine living your own life with being helpful to others, rather than devoting all your energies and efforts to them.

The Negative State

The negative **Centaury** state is characterized by being passive and weak-willed, open to exploitation by others.

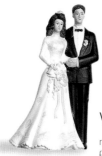

A new start
Walnut is the remedy to take if you are taking a major step forward in life.

WALNUT
According to Dr. Bach, Walnut is the remedy "for those who have decided to take a great step forward in life, to break old conventions, to leave old limits and restrictions, and start on a new way." It is useful for situations in which major changes in life—emotional, spiritual, or even physical, such as moving to a new country—are taking place. Whatever the circumstances, the remedy eases the transition, giving you the confidence to trust in yourself and in your own judgment of what is best for you.

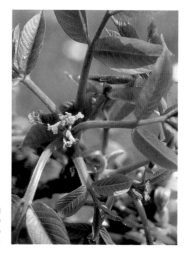

Harvesting
Only female flowers are collected and processed to make the Walnut remedy.

Datafile

BOTANICAL NAME
Juglans regia.

HABITAT
Hedgerows and orchards.

PLANT DESCRIPTION
Walnut trees are massive, rising to a height of about 100 feet (30 meters) when fully mature. Its catkins and flowers—the catkins are male and the flowers female—bloom in mid- to late spring, just before the leaf buds burst or while they are bursting. Only the female flowers, which are less prolific, are used to make the remedy. They grow on their own, or in small groups.

REMEDY PREPARATION
Boiling method. Pick about 6 inches (15 centimeters) of the young shoot, leaves, and female flowers.

INDICATIONS FOR USE
Finding it difficult to make the break and settle down into a new routine, cope with any major change in life and its consequences, or stick to what you have decided to do when confronted by contrary opinions or other disturbing influences.

WHAT TREATMENT SHOULD ACHIEVE
If you have to adjust to a change in your circumstances, lifestyle, or environment, the remedy will encourage you to stick to your decisions once they are made and to stand up for yourself and what you have decided.

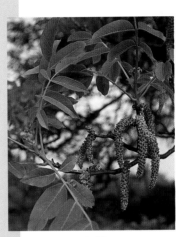

Catkins
Although the catkins are prolific and beautiful only the female flowers are used in the remedy.

The Walnut Remedy

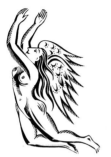

Life changes
Taking Walnut helps people through major changes in life.

Walnut people are usually decisive, at least in theory. Not only do they possess definite ideals and ambitions—they rationalize what they want by setting themselves specific goals that they are determined to achieve.

When it actually comes to the implementation of a decision, however, they can hesitate and become unsure of themselves—and this is exactly when the Walnut remedy comes into play. The link-breaker, as Walnut is sometimes described, is the remedy that helps people to cope with what Dr. Bach called "the big decisions" that inevitably have to be taken in any stage of life. Examples include retirement, having to face the consequences of a major change in lifestyle, or losing a partner or close relative through bereavement. It can also help with weaning, pregnancy, and menopause.

Looking to the future

By helping you to take a step back from factors like outside influences and past preconceptions, the Walnut remedy will help you to approach change positively. With its aid, you will be able to look forward, rather than back. The remedy will stimulate all your positive qualities, such as constancy and determination. As a result, you will remain true to yourself, pursuing what you have decided on without allowing yourself to be thrown off course.

Put at its simplest, Walnut will help you if you find it difficult to break with the past. In addition, it can help you if you are faced with criticism from others. This could be strong enough to make you start to doubt the strength of your convictions, wondering, instead, whether you are making the right move after all. In such circumstances, the Walnut remedy gives you that little bit of extra encouragement you may need to stay the course and see things through to their conclusion.

Learning from Dr. Bach

Some people like to think Dr. Bach himself was a Walnut type. When he abandoned the world of orthodox medicine and its teachings, forsaking all his old ideas to find a better system of healing, he persevered in his endeavors—and eventually triumphed. This was despite the lack of encouragement and, sometimes, the mockery of his former colleagues.

The Negative State

The negative **Walnut** state is characterized by an inability to deal with change and move forward.

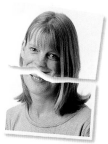

Positive feelings
Holly counters destructive negative emotions.

HOLLY Many Bach practitioners feel that

Holly has a claim to be considered the most important of all the Bach remedies, since it is the antidote for hatred. Holly, as Dr. Bach put it, "protects us from everything that is not Universal Love. Holly opens the heart and unites us with Divine Love." You will find that it will help you if, for whatever reasons, you find yourself totally in the grip of powerful negative emotions directed at another person, such as obsessive jealousy, or a desire to hurt.

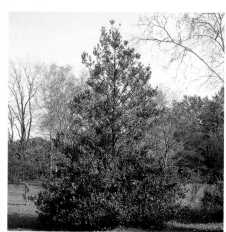

Flowers
Holly's tiny white female flowers bloom in early summer, long before the berries start to appear.

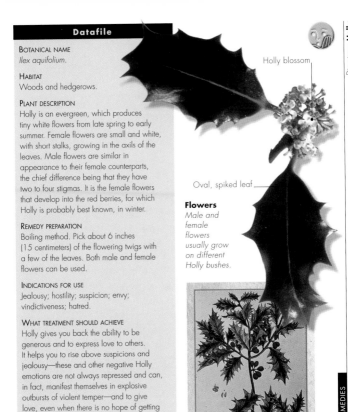

Datafile

BOTANICAL NAME
Ilex aquifolium.

HABITAT
Woods and hedgerows.

PLANT DESCRIPTION
Holly is an evergreen, which produces tiny white flowers from late spring to early summer. Female flowers are small and white, with short stalks, growing in the axils of the leaves. Male flowers are similar in appearance to their female counterparts, the chief difference being that they have two to four stigmas. It is the female flowers that develop into the red berries, for which Holly is probably best known, in winter.

REMEDY PREPARATION
Boiling method. Pick about 6 inches (15 centimeters) of the flowering twigs with a few of the leaves. Both male and female flowers can be used.

INDICATIONS FOR USE
Jealousy; hostility; suspicion; envy; vindictiveness; hatred.

WHAT TREATMENT SHOULD ACHIEVE
Holly gives you back the ability to be generous and to express love to others. It helps you to rise above suspicions and jealousy—these and other negative Holly emotions are not always repressed and can, in fact, manifest themselves in explosive outbursts of violent temper—and to give love, even when there is no hope of getting love in return.

Holly blossom

Oval, spiked leaf

Flowers
Male and female flowers usually grow on different Holly bushes.

Ilex Aquifolium.

The Holly Remedy

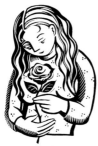

Loving
*Holly gives back the ability
to express love for others.*

If you find that you are developing intensely negative feelings toward others—such as hatred, envy, and the desire to avenge yourself for real or imagined wrongs—then Holly, the remedy of love, will help you to deal with the condition. Otherwise, these negative feelings may cause you considerable emotional and physical suffering, eating you up inside, usually for no good reason.

Taking the Holly remedy will enable you to counter such emotions quickly should they arise, but it is important to

ascertain whether or not it is the appropriate remedy for the specific circumstances. If, for example, you are keeping all your negative feelings firmly bottled up inside you, rather than showing them openly, Willow, rather than Holly, may be a more appropriate choice. This is because it is specifically intended to deal with the inward, unspoken feeling of resentment from which you may be suffering.

Alternatively, if your particular circumstances warrant it, a combination of remedies may be a better alternative. If, say, things have built up to the point where your pent-up feelings start to explode in open outbursts of bad temper, Cherry Plum may be required in addition to Holly. All this means is that you need to think through exactly what your symptoms are indicating.

Analyzing your anger

You need to give a little thought to the reasons for the anger, since anger is a symptom of many different states of mind, each with its own cause or causes. If it is the result of frustration, then a course of Vervain is indicated, and to treat aggression aimed at getting your own way, you should take the Vine remedy.

A last resort

Dr. Bach himself made an interesting observation about Holly and Wild Oat. "If ever a case suggests that it needs many Remedies," he wrote, "or if ever a case does not respond to treatment, give either Holly or Wild Oat, and it will then be obvious which other remedies may be required. In all cases where the patient is of the active, intense type, give Holly. In patients who are of the weak, despondent type, give Wild Oat." This, however, is a last resort. In almost every case, it is sufficient to select the remedies that are needed in the normal way.

The Negative State

The negative **Holly** state is characterized by negative feelings, such as anger, envy, and resentment toward others.

REMEDIES IN ACTION

If you are considering taking the remedies for the first time, you need to be aware from the outset that getting the most out of them involves taking a completely different approach from that of any other healing therapy. Instead of concentrating on physical symptoms and diseases, you need to consider personality and the emotions as the key to cure. The case studies here show how this works in practice.

Case Study

Jenny had suffered two minor car accidents and as a result had developed a fear of driving and become convinced that she would never be safe out on the roads. Even though this was not the case, she was convinced that both accidents were her fault and still felt guilty about them.

Mimulus was suggested, as the remedy for known fears, and **Larch** to deal with Jenny's lack of confidence. **Pine** was advised for her feelings of guilt, plus **White Chestnut** to help her control her worrying thoughts. Finally, **Centaury** was selected to deal with Jenny's propensity to be overanxious to please others. Later, **Mimulus** was discontinued and **Rock Rose** added. Eventually, things improved to the point where Jenny felt able to select her own remedies. Though she will never like driving, she can now drive without fear or panic.

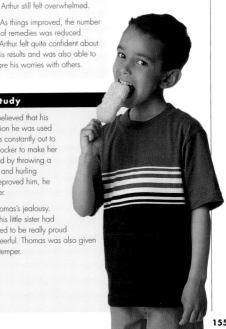

Case Study

Arthur was finding it hard to cope with the thought of his approaching examinations and was extremely tense as a result.

The remedies that were suggested were **Agrimony** to deal with hidden anxieties, **Hornbeam**, for lack of motivation, **Larch** for lack of confidence, **Mimulus** for fear of failure and of letting people down, and **Olive** for tiredness. Later **Elm** was added, since Arthur still felt overwhelmed.

As things improved, the number of remedies was reduced. Arthur felt quite confident about his results and was also able to share his worries with others.

Case Study

Thomas was unhappy because he believed that his baby sister was getting all the attention he was used to receiving from his mother. He was constantly out to attract attention, kicking the baby's rocker to make her cry. If he was scolded, he responded by throwing a temper tantrum, kicking, screaming, and hurling himself onto the floor. If his mother reproved him, he would stamp his feet or try to bite her.

Holly was indicated to deal with Thomas's jealousy. Within a few weeks, his attitude to his little sister had completely changed. He now seemed to be really proud of her, and generally happy and cheerful. Thomas was also given Cherry Plum to help him control his temper.

155

Remedies for Despondency and Despair

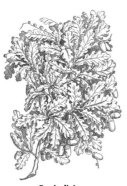

Revitalizing
Oak counters exhaustion and restores lost vitality.

This is the largest of the seven groups of emotional states that Dr. Bach made the cornerstone of his system of healing. It contains eight remedies for eight separate emotional or spiritual states.

Larch is the remedy to take if you lack belief in yourself and your abilities. Pine is indicated if you blame yourself obsessively for everything that goes wrong, regardless of whether or not it is your fault. Put at its simplest, you are weighed down with self-reproach.

Too much to bear

Elm is the remedy of choice for high achievers who suddenly feel they can no longer cope with all the demands being made on them, despite their unquestionable capabilities. Your responsibilities are overwhelming you and you are losing confidence in yourself as a result. Elm helps to restore strength and self-belief. Sweet Chestnut is the remedy to take if you find yourself in a state of utter despair—when things seem so bad that you feel heartbroken as a result. There seems no reason why the darkness into which you have been plunged should ever lift—for you, there is not the vaguest glimmer of light at the end of the tunnel. Star of Bethlehem is the remedy for shock and its after-effects. It will help you to deal with a sudden shock, such as someone dying unexpectedly; it is also an invaluable standby if the trauma surfaces long after the event. Willow will help if you are wrapped up in self-pity. You may see yourself as the plaything of fate, feeling that whatever is happening to you is not your fault. Oak people, in contrast, are usually extremely positive. Sometimes, though, they overtax their strength, in which case the remedy helps to recharge their batteries. Crab Apple is a "cleansing remedy." Dr. Bach described it as the remedy "which helps us to get rid of anything we do not like either in our minds or our bodies."

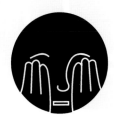

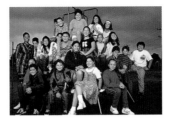

Confidence
Taking Larch gives you the courage you need to try to succeed.

LARCH
A lack of self-confidence is characteristic of Larch people. They doubt their abilities, and their feelings of insecurity may be so pronounced that they are convinced that anything they try to accomplish will end in failure. Taking the remedy, however, will help them to be able to assess objectives realistically and learn how to pursue success, rather than always looking on the negative side and getting accustomed to expectations of failure.

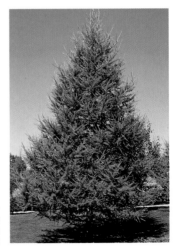

Deciduous conifer
Larch in full leaf. It is the only conifer to shed its leaves in winter completely.

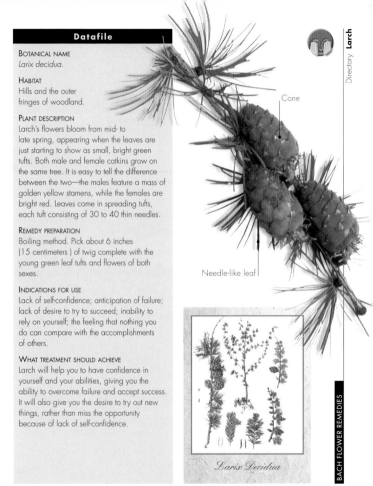

Datafile

BOTANICAL NAME
Larix decidua.

HABITAT
Hills and the outer
fringes of woodland.

PLANT DESCRIPTION
Larch's flowers bloom from mid- to
late spring, appearing when the leaves are
just starting to show as small, bright green
tufts. Both male and female catkins grow on
the same tree. It is easy to tell the difference
between the two—the males feature a mass of
golden yellow stamens, while the females are
bright red. Leaves come in spreading tufts,
each tuft consisting of 30 to 40 thin needles.

REMEDY PREPARATION
Boiling method. Pick about 6 inches
(15 centimeters) of twig complete with the
young green leaf tufts and flowers of both
sexes.

INDICATIONS FOR USE
Lack of self-confidence; anticipation of failure;
lack of desire to try to succeed; inability to
rely on yourself; the feeling that nothing you
do can compare with the accomplishments
of others.

WHAT TREATMENT SHOULD ACHIEVE
Larch will help you to have confidence in
yourself and your abilities, giving you the
ability to overcome failure and accept success.
It will also give you the desire to try out new
things, rather than miss the opportunity
because of lack of self-confidence.

Cone

Needle-like leaf

Larix Decidua

The Larch Remedy

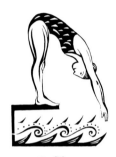

Confidence
*Larch gives you the confidence
to take the plunge into life.*

If you are in a negative Larch state, your lack of self-confidence means that you have resigned yourself to failure from the word go. You have managed to convince yourself that there are all sorts of things that you just cannot tackle and your answer to the problem is simply to avoid even attempting to face it. What this means, of course, is that you are depriving yourself of opportunities.

The reasons why you cannot or will not undertake certain things seem completely rational, at least as far as

you are concerned. The lack of confidence that lies behind it all may stem back to childhood experiences—or earlier, since there is a view that such feelings may well be passed down the chain from one generation to another.

However, the problem more often than not is a temporary one, arising particularly at times when you are likely to be suffering from some degree of stress as well. The remedy is effective in handling pre-examination nerves, as well as helping people to cope with, for instance, job interviews.

From failure to success

Rather than expecting to fail due to your lack of self-confidence, the remedy will help you to transform your attitude to life and all the opportunities it has to offer, which you are currently passing up. It does this by removing the fear of failure, which, in itself, stems from lack of confidence in yourself and in your ability to succeed in whatever you have set out to do. You will come to realize that you are not only equally capable but may even be more capable than others, including your rivals and competitors.

Now you have allowed your true potential to come forward and express itself, you will find that you have the ability to take the initiative, rather than always waiting on events. Your approach to life will change as well, now that you have the confidence to take a more relaxed view of things. As a result, you will be able to get far more out of life, learning how to maximize its opportunities rather than letting them by-pass you as you did previously.

You will learn how to take advantage of Dr. Bach's advice to "plunge into life." Without this, "we shall learn but little," even though the reason that we are here is to "gain experience and knowledge."

The Negative State

The negative **Larch State** is characterized by a lack of self-confidence, insecurity and an expectation of failure.

Guilt complex
*Pine puts you straight if you
are obsessed with feelings
of guilt that are unjustified.*

PINE
With or without cause, Pine people feel guilty and full of self-reproach. People in a negative Pine state always seem to be apologizing and take every opportunity to punish themselves for their supposed failings. The remedy is a lifeline that gives them the ability to differentiate the wood from the trees, enabling them to determine which errors they are responsible for and which they are not, so they feel genuine regret and only when it is appropriate for them to do so.

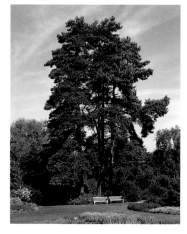

Flowers
*Both male and
female flowers are
needed to produce
the Pine remedy.*

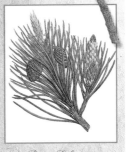

Datafile

BOTANICAL NAME
Pinus sylvestris.

HABITAT
Pine woods and heathland, preferring sandy soil.

PLANT DESCRIPTION
The male and female flowers grow on the same tree, blossoming in late spring and early summer. The male flowers, which are golden yellow, form clusters at the top of the shorter shoots; the egg-shaped red female cones grow singly, or in clusters of three, at the shoot's apex.

REMEDY PREPARATION
Boiling method. Pick about 6 inches (15 centimeters) of the young shoots, together with both male and female flowers, when the male flowers are in full pollen.

INDICATIONS FOR USE
Self-reproach; plagued by feelings of guilt and unworthiness; taking the blame for the guilt of others; dwelling on past mistakes; incessantly analyzing your own actions and finding yourself at fault.

WHAT TREATMENT SHOULD ACHIEVE
If you are in a negative Pine state, you are drowning in a sea of guilt. Taking the Pine remedy will help you reach the shore in safety. It is a lifebelt that helps you face up to errors and apologize for them only when they really are your responsibility. It also helps you to stop apologizing for yourself constantly, even when there is absolutely no need to do so.

Leaf tufts surround flowerheads

Small flexible branches lead off the main ones

Pinus Sylvestris

The Pine Remedy

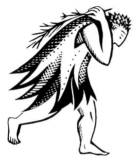

Apologetic
*Pine people use
guilt as a rod for their
own backs.*

Pine people feel perpetually guilty. They will carry on blaming themselves for anything and everything, even if it is obvious to outsiders that they have nothing to feel guilty about, since they have done absolutely nothing wrong. Their favorite word is undoubtedly "sorry."

If you are in a negative Pine state, your first inclination is to blame yourself for anything that goes wrong and immediately to start apologizing for it, even if the fault lies elsewhere. The state need not be the result of something immediate; it can be triggered by a past event, which has been buried, but now comes to the surface.

There is even more to the problem than this, however. If you are in this sort of emotional black hole, you are probably never really satisfied with what you achieve. This may lead you to overwork and will certainly contribute to your emotional stress.

Making yourself a scapegoat

Nor will you be getting much pleasure out of life to compensate for this, since you are only too willing to accept the role of the natural scapegoat, constantly apologizing for yourself even when there is no need for you to do so. Even in a casual conversation, for instance, apologetic turns of phrase will keep appearing—a habit that applies to practically every other situation in which you might find yourself. What you are doing is unconsciously undermining yourself, thanks to a negative self-image, which nothing and nobody appear able to change. Instead, you will constantly undervalue yourself and your abilities, and fail to recognize your achievements.

Putting things in perspective

With the help of the Pine remedy, however, life can be transformed. It has the same effect as that of recharging a flat battery—it gives you the boost you need to realize that there are natural limits to blame and responsibility.

Though you will still be able to acknowledge errors, now it will be only the ones for which you are actually responsible. You will no longer be looking for a rod for your own back. This total change in attitude will influence the whole of your life for the better, particularly as far as your relationships with others are concerned.

The Negative State

The negative **Pine** state is characterized by unfounded feelings of guilt and dissatisfaction with your achievements.

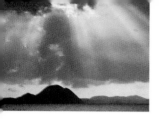

Overburdened
Elm people can find the sudden inability to cope traumatic, just like a storm arising out of a clear sky.

ELM

It is likely that Elm people will be successful high achievers, but they may face problems nevertheless. These stem from their tendency to take on too many commitments. As a result, they suffer from bouts of depression when they feel unable to cope with so many self-imposed tasks. The remedy helps by calming their minds, giving them the chance to regain the confidence to deal with problems rationally, rather than giving way to the feeling of being overwhelmed, with all the negative consequences this may entail.

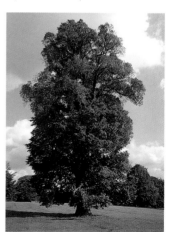

Dutch Elm disease
Elm is rarer now than it used to be as a result of Dutch Elm disease.

Datafile

BOTANICAL NAME
Ulmus procera.

HABITAT
Woodlands and hedgerows.

PLANT DESCRIPTION
The elm tree has a massive trunk, deeply fissured grayish bark, and many spreading branches. The small and numerous purplish-brown flowers, which grow in clusters, blossom from late winter to midspring, opening before the leaves.

REMEDY PREPARATION
Boiling method. Pick about 6 inches (15 centimeters) of twig with the flower clusters.

INDICATIONS FOR USE
Temporary feelings of inadequacy and lack of self-confidence; being overwhelmed by your responsibilities; bouts of despondency and exhaustion caused by taking on too much.

WHAT TREATMENT SHOULD ACHIEVE
Elm will help you to recover your self-confidence and give you the ability to see problems in perspective. Responsible, reliable, and self-assured, you will now be able to assume the burdens of responsibility without flinching from them, since you will be confident that help is at hand when you need it.

Leaves
Elm leaves open on the bare twigs once the flowers have bloomed.

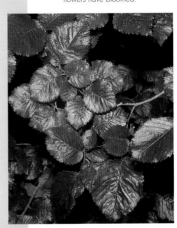

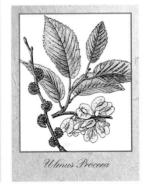

Ulmus Procera

The Elm Remedy

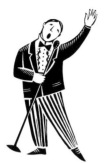

Self-confidence
*Elm people are high
achievers who
welcome responsibility.*

If, at times, you find yourself feeling overwhelmed by responsibilities, the Elm remedy is there ready to come to your rescue. Such feelings are always unpleasant, no matter what type of person you are, but for Elm people they can be even more traumatic than usual.

This is because Elm types, on the whole, are capable and efficient. They are high achievers, who come close to being indispensable in whatever capacity they fulfill. Almost invariably, they are responsible for others, who are

dependent on what they decide. Their weakness is their willingness to take on more and more, a process that may carry on escalating until something simply has to give under the strain.

The Elm crisis

The crisis breaks, when, at a crucial moment, such people suddenly start to feel that there is no way that they can possibly satisfy all the demands that are being made on them, even though it is likely that at least some of these demands are self-imposed. As a result of this realization, they may lapse into a state of dejection or even start to suffer from depression.

The simple fact is that, despite their best efforts, they now are afraid of being unable to cope with the number of responsibilities that they have accumulated. These feelings can be made worse by the realization that others are depending on them.

Fortunately, it is rare for this negative state to last for long, since Elm people's underlying confidence means that they are usually quick to recover their poise and stability. A lot of this comes from the conviction that they have found their calling. When it comes down to it, this makes them sure that, somewhere within themselves, they will be able to find the extra strength that they need in order to complete all the various duties and tasks that they have undertaken.

How the remedy helps

Taking the remedy obviously helps in reestablishing the status quo, especially if things have reached a point where your underlying confidence in your abilities has been temporarily negated. Its effects can be almost immediate, quickly countering the belief that your tasks have grown beyond your ability to deal with them. You will rapidly recover your spirits, together with the self-belief that is the key to success.

The Negative State

The negative **Elm** state is characterized by dejection and depression caused by being overwhelmed by responsibilities.

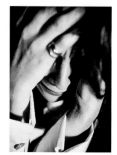

Anguish
Sweet Chestnut helps to relieve extreme cases of mental and physical suffering.

SWEET CHESTNUT If you
are in a negative Sweet Chestnut state, you will be suffering unbearable anguish. Literally, you will be at the end of your tether, unable to break free of the ever-tightening chains that are confining you, or to cope with the pain and suffering the state involves. Taking the remedy gives you the crucial injection of hope you need to battle on. It will help to relieve your heartache and show you that there is no final defeat.

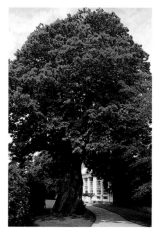

Late-blossoming
Sweet Chestnut is a deciduous tree which is relatively late to blossom.

Datafile

BOTANICAL NAME
Castanea sativa.

HABITAT
Open woodland.

PLANT DESCRIPTION
The remedy comes from the flowers of the Spanish, or Edible, Chestnut, which bloom from early to late summer. Both male and female catkins, which grow on the same tree, are long, slender, and pale yellow in color. The lower ones are predominantly male; their pollen has a sickly scent when it is ripe. The upper, female ones are fewer in number, growing in clusters of two or three.

REMEDY PREPARATION
Boiling method. Pick about 6 inches (15 centimeters) of twig complete with leaves and male and female flowers.

INDICATIONS FOR USE
Feelings of absolute dejection; deep mental anguish and despair; believing that you have reached the limits of endurance; feeling lost and empty inside; abandoning all hope; fearing a complete mental and physical breakdown.

WHAT TREATMENT SHOULD ACHIEVE
Sweet Chestnut helps when everything is hopeless and there is no way out. Once again, you will be able to see light at the end of the tunnel and your faith and hope will be restored.

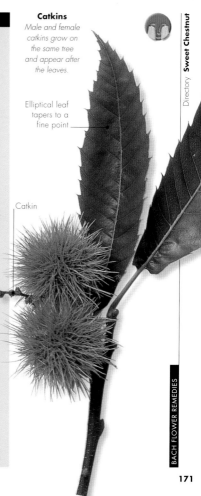

Catkins
Male and female catkins grow on the same tree and appear after the leaves.

Elliptical leaf tapers to a fine point

Catkin

The Sweet Chestnut Remedy

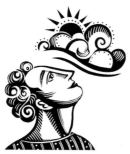

A glimmer of hope

*Sweet Chestnut provides hope
in cases of utter despair.*

Sweet Chestnut, wrote Dr. Bach in *The Twelve Healers and Other Remedies*, is the one [remedy] "for that terrible, that appalling mental despair when it seems the very soul itself is suffering destruction. It is the hopeless despair of those who feel they have reached the limit of their endurance."

In a negative Sweet Chestnut state, your back will be against the wall. You have reached the point where, though you have battled on and on regardless, you have hit rock bottom and you simply cannot take any more. Even the people closest to you cannot help: there is no way out of the pit in which you are trapped. The despair can be so acute that you may turn to thinking of death (though you may doubt whether even that will put an end to your sufferings). In extremes, you may even begin to think that you are in danger of going insane, or suffering a major mental breakdown.

Relying on faith

The remedy can help you by promoting your sense of personal faith, for, as Dr. Bach said, "this is the moment when miracles are done." It was a faith that he himself certainly possessed in abundance, as he demonstrated when he "called in the profession" to save his colleagues "from trouble, complications, inquests, and so on" just before his death. Though, of course, we cannot tell what his exact feelings were at this time, it is more than likely that he was not afraid of death, since his personal faith in the power of providence was so strong. Dr. Bach was remembering how he had been given up for dead in 1917 by his colleagues: God had allowed him nearly two decades more of life for the purpose of completing his allotted tasks on Earth.

Offering hope

The remedy will help you to cope with despair and desolation: it will also give you renewed hope that, despite appearances, the state may prove to be a transitory one and better times may be ahead. Sometimes, though, a sense of acceptance and faith may be all that can be provided, since there may truly be no complete solution to the problem.

The Negative State

The negative **Sweet Chestnut** state is characterized by absolute dejection, despair, mental anguish, and total exhaustion.

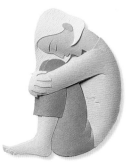

Shock antidote
The Star of Bethlehem remedy can help to counter shock and its after-effects.

STAR OF BETHLEHEM

Star of Bethlehem is one of the five remedies that Dr. Bach included in his Rescue Remedy, its function being to neutralize shock and its after-effects. For instance, Star of Bethlehem on its own will help you to cope with bad news, or with the effects of an accident either yourself, or on someone close to you. It is also the remedy to turn to in cases of delayed shock (which can manifest itself long after the original event).

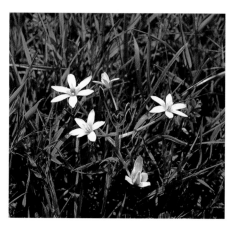

Bulb
Like garlic, Star of Bethlehem starts off its life as a bulb.

Datafile

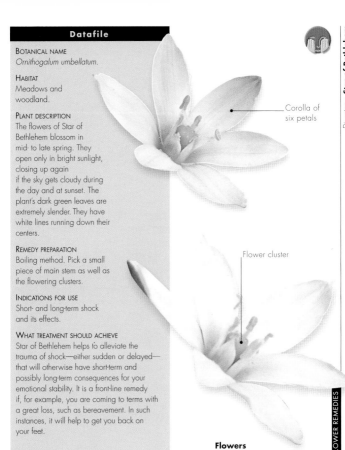

BOTANICAL NAME
Ornithogalum umbellatum.

HABITAT
Meadows and
woodland.

PLANT DESCRIPTION
The flowers of Star of
Bethlehem blossom in
mid- to late spring. They
open only in bright sunlight,
closing up again
if the sky gets cloudy during
the day and at sunset. The
plant's dark green leaves are
extremely slender. They have
white lines running down their
centers.

REMEDY PREPARATION
Boiling method. Pick a small
piece of main stem as well as
the flowering clusters.

INDICATIONS FOR USE
Short- and long-term shock
and its effects.

WHAT TREATMENT SHOULD ACHIEVE
Star of Bethlehem helps to alleviate the
trauma of shock—either sudden or delayed—
that will otherwise have short-term and
possibly long-term consequences for your
emotional stability. It is a front-line remedy
if, for example, you are coming to terms with
a great loss, such as bereavement. In such
instances, it will help to get you back on
your feet.

Corolla of
six petals

Flower cluster

Flowers
*The star-shaped white
flowers are striped
with green.*

The Star of Bethlehem Remedy

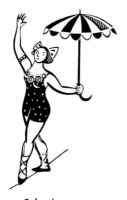

Balancing
Star of Bethlehem helps you remain balanced in case of shock.

example of a situation in which the remedy is of use is in the case of a bereavement. In this situation, the remedy will ease the pain of parting, helping you to come to terms with grief. Many bereaved people need all the help they can get to stop them from breaking down completely. This is not to be confused with having a good cry, which may be just what they needed.

Unlocking the emotions

Star of Bethlehem is particularly useful if, for whatever reason, you are bottling up your emotions, rather than giving vent to your feelings. As any psychologist or counselor will tell you, this is extremely counterproductive, since ultimately it can only make the situation worse.

The remedy is the key to unlocking these pent-up emotions, helping to relieve all the pressures that would otherwise be building up inside you. In addition to this, it can also help you to cope with any physical side effects of,

Dr. Bach described Star of Bethlehem as "the comforter and soother of pains and sorrows." It is the remedy of first choice when it comes to treating any case of severe shock or trauma. Star of Bethlehem will help you if you are involved in a road accident, for instance, but there is a host of other possible triggers. A classic for example, an injury that has sparked off the initial shock, since, once emotions are stabilized, the body can bounce back to its natural state of health.

Dealing with delayed shock

Sometimes, the effects of shock do not show themselves immediately. Instead, they are repressed, lurking in the background until they come to the surface. This can take weeks, months, or even years, long after the original incident has been forgotten. In such instances, the shock may reveal itself as any one of a number of physical or mental ailments with no apparent cause. In such instances, Star of Bethlehem can still help to resolve the after-effects of shock even many years after the event.

The Negative State

The negative **Star of Bethlehem** state is characterized by being in severe turmoil after a shock or trauma.

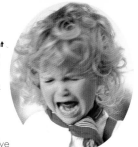

WILLOW

People in a negative Willow state are packed full of self-pity, believing that everything always goes wrong for them through no fault of their own. Rather, it is other people—or sometimes even life itself—that are conspiring against them and so are always to blame. Nothing is ever their fault. Like a dormant volcano, they smolder with resentment, although it never comes to a full-scale eruption. A course of Willow will help reawaken the ability to look on the positive side, rather than always approaching things from a negative standpoint. They will discover that they, too, can have a more optimistic attitude to life.

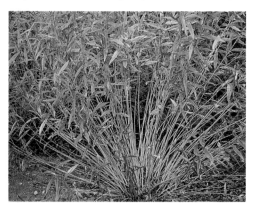

Catkins

Long, slender catkins emerge at the same time as the leaves unfold.

Datafile

BOTANICAL NAME
Salix vitellina.

HABITAT
Moist, low-lying ground.

PLANT DESCRIPTION
S. vitellina (the Golden Osier
or Yellow Willow) is the only
Willow variety that can be used
to make the Willow remedy.
You can recognize it by its twigs,
which are brilliant yellow in
winter. In late spring, when
S. vitellina blooms, long, slender
male and female catkins appear.

REMEDY PREPARATION
Boiling method. You will need
male and female catkins, the
young leaves, and about
6 inches (15 centimeters) of twig.

INDICATIONS FOR USE
Resentfulness; bitterness; self-pity;
the belief that you have been and
are being treated unfairly;
blaming others for what is
happening to you; lack of
fulfillment; the feeling that you are
not getting what you deserve;
never-ending carping and
complaining about anything
and everything.

WHAT TREATMENT SHOULD ACHIEVE
Taking the remedy will help you to feel less
bitter. Instead, you will be more optimistic
about life, and come to see just what
friendship and companionship both
have to offer you.

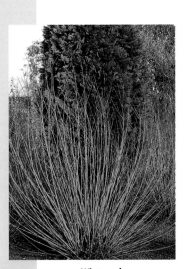

Winter color
*The Golden Osier gets
its name from the fact
that it turns bright
yellow in winter.*

The Willow Remedy

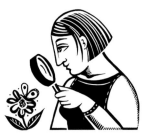

Looking outward
*Willow people are
introspective and full
of self-pity.*

Willow people have turned in on themselves, becoming extremely negative in their thinking as a result. They can never see the good in anything, but one thing that they are certain of is that nothing is their fault. Whatever the situation, they are the first to put a damper on things, with the result that they come across to others as being the proverbial wet blankets and spoilsports. If you are in a negative Willow state, the chances are that you feel victimized, unjustly treated by life,

and full of bitterness and resentment. Morose, moody, touchy, and resentful, you begrudge others any good fortune and, although you expect a great deal from life, you are not prepared to put anything back in return.

You are ungrateful, too, being prepared to accept advice and help as a matter of course, but the last thing you would see the need to do is to express any thanks in return. In the long term, this leads to your alienating others, who simply have no more patience with your selfish self-pity. The isolation that is almost an inevitable consequence only makes matters worse, since it encourages you to be even more resentful, as you withdraw into your shell more and more.

Getting out of the pit

If you find yourself in this position, the first thing you have to realize is that you—and you alone—are responsible for the state of mind into which you have fallen. You have to stop perpetually looking inward and take steps to break down the invisible barriers with which you have surrounded yourself. This is what the Willow remedy helps you to do. It is important that you do something, otherwise the state can progress from being a temporary to a permanent one. If this happens, you will find that all the self-pity, resentment, and self-regard start to feed off one another to make matters even worse.

Taking the remedy helps you to throw off the negative chains that hitherto have been keeping you firmly in the toils. You will now find it possible to be generous about other people, rather then resenting them and their efforts, appreciating and learning from them. At the same time, you will come to realize that, although you may find it hard to believe it at first, it is possible that you are not always right and are quite capable of getting something wrong.

The Negative State

The negative **Willow** state is characterized by feelings of bitterness and resentment, and always seeing the negative side of things.

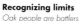

Recognizing limits
Oak people are battlers who can exhaust their energy reserves.

OAK

Oak people are extremely positive in their approach to life. They are fighters who never lose hope or give up. Any problems they have stem from their tendency to draw constantly on their internal strengths, ignoring Nature's alarm signals and exhausting even their massive energy reserves as a result. The Oak remedy helps with this problem in two ways. As well as recharging your batteries, it will help you to recognize that there are limits even to your strength, and that there is a time to rest.

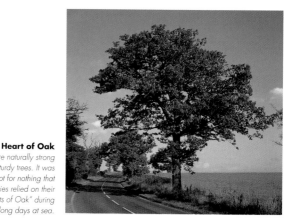

Heart of Oak
Oaks are naturally strong and sturdy trees. It was not for nothing that navies relied on their "Hearts of Oak" during their long days at sea.

Datafile

BOTANICAL NAME
Quercus robur.

HABITAT
Woods, hedgerows, and meadows.

PLANT DESCRIPTION
Male and female flowers develop on the same tree, blossoming in mid- to late spring at the same time that the young leaves start to emerge. The male catkins, which are yellowish in color, come in loose, drooping clusters. The tiny scarlet-tipped female flowers, which are far less numerous, are usually hidden in groups of two to five among the new leaves.

REMEDY PREPARATION
Sun method.

INDICATIONS FOR USE
Feeling utterly worn out and exhausted in mind, body, and spirit, but carrying on and never complaining about it; ignoring natural impulses to rest; endeavoring not to let tiredness and weakness show; making hard, methodical efforts beyond the limits of your strength.

WHAT TREATMENT SHOULD ACHIEVE
By recharging your internal batteries, the remedy will help to give you the renewed strength to overcome all life's vicissitudes. It will also help to replenish and enhance qualities of endurance, reliability, steadfastness, and common sense. You will be able to set reasonable limits to your efforts, and allow yourself time to rest.

Remedy
Only the female flowers are used in the preparation of the Oak remedy.

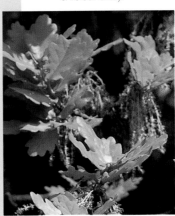

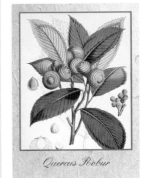

Quercus Robur

The Oak Remedy

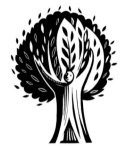

Strength
Like the Oak tree, Oak people are strong and sturdy.

Oak people, like the tree itself, are extremely strong physically and mentally. They are reliable, dependable, patient, and full of common sense. Even more to the point, they are never prepared to give up hope whatever the nature or seriousness of the problems that life may confront them with from time to time. As Dr. Bach put it, "They are brave people, fighting against great difficulties without loss of hope or slackening of effort." What this means in practice is that even if things become too much for you, with your reserves of energy all but exhausted, you will struggle on against all the odds without complaint. Indeed, you will try to conceal the fact that you may be tired and feeling down from all those around you, because you are not prepared to let anything interfere with the fulfillment of whatever it is that you have set out to accomplish.

If the pressure continues unabated, however, even your considerable willpower, devotion to your duty, and almost superhuman powers of endurance may no longer be enough. Even the most resilient Oak person can reach a point where he or she cracks.

Recognizing the danger point

If you are in any danger of reaching this point, you need to take remedial action quickly. There comes a definite time when simply battling on and on is counterproductive, since it is now becoming an end in itself rather than a means to an end. Regardless of any outward appearances, you are suffering within yourself, and the problem, if left unresolved, can only go from bad to worse. There is no obvious way out of the situation either, since it is a cornerstone of your creed to carry on regardless and never to let others down. It is likely that they have come to depend on you precisely because of your positive qualities, particularly your reliability.

Learning to give and take

This is where the Oak remedy can help by encouraging you to become more flexible in your approach. As well as helping you to recover your lost vitality and rekindle your zest for life and living, you now will become aware of the fact that there are limits even to your strength. You cannot go on regardless for ever and ever—you must make the time to take a step back from what you are doing to rest and relax.

The Negative State

The negative **Oak** state is characterized by plodding on with life to the point of physical and mental exhaustion.

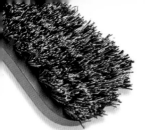

CRAB APPLE

Recognized by all Bach practitioners as the "cleansing" remedy, Crab Apple should be taken if you ever feel physically soiled—as a result, for instance, of illness and disease, pollution, or simply touching something that is dirty. You should also take it if you feel mentally unclean, especially if you are suffering from feelings of self-disgust and self-loathing. It will also help if you are suffering from obsessive behavior, or are overconcentrating on minor details at the expense of more important things.

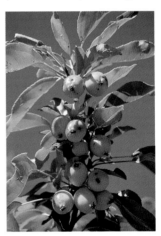

Fruit
The fruit of the Crab Apple grows in clusters at the end of dwarf spurs.

Datafile

BOTANICAL NAME
Malus pumila.

HABITAT
Hedges, thickets and open woodland.

PLANT DESCRIPTION
Crab Apple blooms in late spring. Its pretty, heart-shaped flowers are a rich pink on the outside and pink with a touch of white within. They are relatively easy to gather, since they grow in clusters. on dwarf spurs.

REMEDY PREPARATION
Boiling method. Pick the flowers on their spurs, together with their leaves.

INDICATIONS FOR USE
Feeling physically or mentally unclean; finding fault with your appearance; getting bogged down in details; obsessive behavior of any type.

WHAT TREATMENT SHOULD ACHIEVE
Crab Apple works by encouraging you to appreciate all your positive qualities, rather than becoming obsessed with negative ones. It will help you to resolve the inner disharmony from which you may be suffering.

Flowers
Crab Apple's flowers are a rich pink on the outside with a touch of white in the centre.

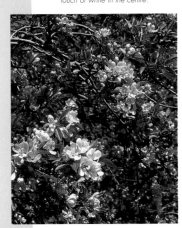

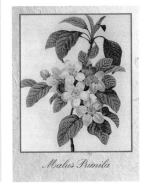

Malus Pumila

The Crab Apple Remedy

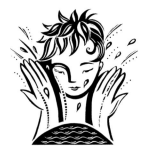

Purgative
*Crab Apple purges
uncleanliness from
mind and body.*

Crab Apple has a specific role of healing in the Bach system. It is the remedy you should turn to if, for whatever reason, you feel soiled, dirty, or unclean.

Sometimes, the trigger for such feelings can be physical—an outbreak of eczema, the appearance of an unsightly rash, warts, acne, and other skin complaints, and moles have all been known to spark off negative Crab Apple states. So, too, may negative behavior patterns—if, for instance, you find yourself deliberately being unkind. It can also be triggered by self-disgust at your own bad habits, which, despite all your efforts, you find impossible to break, however much you know within yourself that you ought to make a determined effort to crack them. Classic examples of this include smoking, especially if you are a reformed smoker who has lapsed, and drinking too much, too often.

Another clear indication of a negative Crab Apple state is becoming obsessed with triviality. You cannot see the wood for the trees, falling victim to the temptation of getting bogged down in detail—sometimes at the expense of things that common sense would seem to indicate should be far more important.

Taking the remedy

Crab Apple will help you to cope with all these problems. Indeed, some Bach practitioners would argue that the recognition that there is a problem that ought to be tackled in the first place is a clear sign that you are already taking the first steps that will lead to its eventual resolution. What it does is to help you to regain control of your patterns of thought, giving you the wisdom to see things in perspective. Rather than dwelling on trifles to the point of obsessiveness, you will gain broad-mindedness. Even more importantly, you will realize that you have been suffering from something that you have the power within yourself to rectify.

Depending on circumstances, there are various ways you can actually take the remedy, so you should choose the one that is most suited to your particular needs. You can take drops as you would do normally. In addition, you can use it as a lotion—or, if you prefer, as a compress—if there are physical symptoms. You could try adding it to a bath—six drops are ample for the average-sized bathtub.

The Negative State

The negative **Crab Apple** state is characterized by feelings of being unclean, shame, and self-disgust.

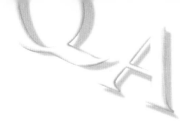

QUESTIONS & ANSWERS

Bach practitioners positively welcome it when people ask questions about Dr. Bach, the remedies he discovered, and the system of healing of which they form an integral part. What Dr. Bach created was a self-help system. Good practitioners will encourage you to find out more about the remedies, so that you can use them for yourself. A further starting point is Dr. Bach's last book—*The Twelve Healers and Other Remedies*—in which he set down his final, perfected thoughts on the 38 remedies he had discovered.

Q While I was taking the remedies, I developed a throat infection. Did this happen as a result of taking the remedy?

A *Very rarely, people using the remedies report mild physical symptoms. These are part of the cleansing process and nothing at all to worry about. If the* symptoms were serious, the chances are that this was a coincidence. Your health can only be improved as a result of the balance the remedies will bring.

Q How long do the remedies last?

A *The use-by date on the stock bottles refers to the shelf-life of the alcohol content and is a legal requirement. Experience shows that the remedies themselves retain their potency indefinitely.*

Q My problem is that I see a little of myself in almost all the negative characteristics of the various remedy descriptions. How do I find which remedies I really need? Are there specific ones with which to start?

A *There is no pecking order of remedies, although some, like Olive and White Chestnut, are more commonly needed than, say, Rock Water and Water Violet. The thing to do is to think about the way you are feeling and, if more than seven remedies seem indicated, cross out the ones that relate to passing moods. Remember, the effort of thinking about yourself and the way you are feeling is therapeutic in itself.*

Q I accept that the remedies contain the life essence of the flowers themselves, but I don't understand what this is. Nor do I understand how the remedies work. Can you help me?

A *No doubt one day the active ingredient will be isolated, but, at present, the only true answer is to say that people talk about abstracts like "subtle energy" and vibrations, but the best definition is still Dr. Bach's own. He compared them to beautiful music, which makes you feel happier and better, although you don't know why it should.*

Q How long do I have to take the remedies before I can expect to start seeing the results?

A *It depends on how deep the problem actually is. Sometimes, they can act very quickly, but you should expect to see to some improvement after three weeks.*

Q Can Bach remedies be used with other remedies?

A *Yes. While Bach flower remedies can be thought of as a complete system of healing, they are also safe to use as an adjunct to other complementary or conventional therapies.*

Remedies for Overanxiety for Others' Welfare

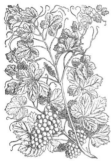

Vine
Vine people can be very domineering and uncompromising.

The last group of emotional states Dr. Bach identified contains five remedies, all of which deal with various forms of selfishness.

Chicory, for instance, is the remedy you need if you have a tendency to be overpossessive. People in this state tend to be egocentric, determined to achieve their own ends. If they do not get their own way, they do not keep quiet about it. Instead, they proclaim their woes from the rooftops—indeed, they can even be brought to tears by what they feel is the ingratitude that others are showing toward them for all their effort.

Imposing the will

Vervain people are strongly opinionated and set in their ways—they, too, seek to impose their views and ideas on others. They are often their own worst enemies, since they can easily fall victim to over enthusiasm. If this is not brought back into check, it can spur them on to try harder and harder, and eventually overtax their mental and physical strength.

Vine people are similarly strong willed. They are also ambitious. However, they can fall victim to the temptation to exploit their gifts for the purposes of domination, tending to ride roughshod over people as a result. This stems from their absolute conviction that they are always in the right. Beech people are critics, quick to condemn anything that they do not understand, rather than trying to come to terms with others' points of view. Their intolerance can make them irritable and bad-tempered.

Finally, there is the Rock Water type. In contrast to Vine people, Rock Water people, as a rule, do not try to meddle in other people's lives. Rather, they have turned in on themselves. Full of high ideals, but rigid and inflexible, they can become their own harshest critics as they try to live up to the extremely high standards they have set for themselves.

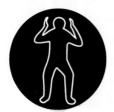

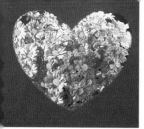

Demanding
Chicory people may seem all heart, but, in the negative state, they can be extremely selfish and demanding.

CHICORY
On the surface at least, Chicory people may seem selfless, since it appears that they are devoting time and energy to worrying about others. In fact, they are overpossessive, constantly prying into the lives of those close to them. If this leads to rejection, self-pity can take a hold, since they cannot see why their attentions are not appreciated. Taking the remedy helps people with these problems show true concern for others.

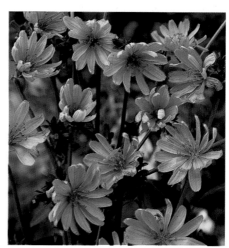

Flowers
Chicory blooms in high summer. Only a few flowers emerge at a time.

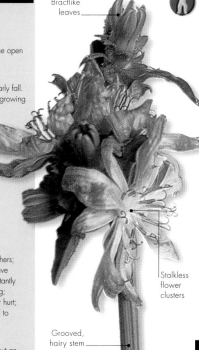

Datafile

BOTANICAL NAME
Chichorium intybus.

HABITAT
Gravel, chalky soil, wasteland, and the open borders of roadsides and fields.

PLANT DESCRIPTION
Chicory blooms from midsummer to early fall. The blue starlike flowers are stalkless, growing in clusters of two or three flowers each in the axils of the stem-leaves.

REMEDY PREPARATION
Sun method. The flowers are extremely delicate, the result being that they fade quickly when picked. For this reason, it is best to pick only two or three flowers at a time, floating them quickly on the surface of the water.

INDICATIONS FOR USE
Demanding time and attention from others; holding on to emotional bonds that have had their day; taking pleasure in constantly commenting, correcting, and criticizing; feeling easily slighted, passed over, or hurt; growing angry and resentful if you fail to receive love and attention.

WHAT TREATMENT SHOULD ACHIEVE
The remedy works by helping you to put an end to selfishness and selfish desires. Instead, you will be able to give love and devotion to others without expecting or needing anything in return. You will feel more secure in yourself as a result.

Bractlike leaves

Stalkless flower clusters

Grooved, hairy stem

Delicate
Flowers should be used quickly, they soon start to fade once picked.

The Chicory Remedy

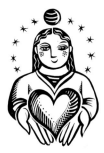

Caring
*The remedy will help
you to show genuine
concern for others.*

At their most positive, Chicory people are wonderful, caring friends and parents. However, there is a darker obverse side to the Chicory state. At their most negative, although this is an extreme situation, such people can be emotional leeches.

In such circumstances, although people in a negative Chicory state give the surface impression that their sole aim is to ensure the happiness and well-being of others, the reality is somewhat different. Chicory devotion can be

extremely selfish and cloying, stemming not from any altruistic concerns, but rather the product of possessiveness and self-concern.

You may find, for instance, that people in a negative Chicory state are prone to bringing up the notion of "duty" in conversation: the last thing they mean by this, though, is the duty they might owe to others. On the contrary, what they mean is the duty owed to them. They expect constant gratitude and praise, and, if this is not forthcoming, they become full of self-pity and even tearful in response to what they believe is lack of appreciation.

Dealing with selfishness

Children in a negative Chicory state are basically unhappy and need help. Otherwise, their problems can put pressure on the close, loving relationship that should exist between parent and child. At any age, though, the state should not be left untreated. If you come under the influence of a Chicory person, you will soon know all

about it. You may find is that your own
energy is being sapped by the demands
they will be making on you. Not only
will a great deal be expected of you,
as if by right, what you may also find is
that it is hard to break free without
being emotionally affected yourself.

The Chicory transformation
The outlook is by no means totally
bleak, since there is always the
potential to take advantage of the
undoubted capacity for love and
affection that is characteristic of a
positive Chicory state. The remedy sows
the seeds for this transformation. When
it happens, you will find that it
is possible for you to be selfless rather
than selfish, gaining the ability to give
without expecting anything in return.
As a result, you will feel far happier
within yourself.

The Negative State

The negative **Chicory** state is characterized by
selfishness, possessiveness, and egotistic self-
concern combined with dominating others.

197

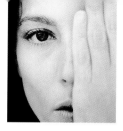

VERVAIN

As Dr. Bach noted, Vervain people are often full of "big ideals and ambitions for the good of humanity," they "do not like to listen to advice" and can be "intolerant of the opinions of others." They are strong-willed and problems arise if they get carried away with their own enthusiasm, when their inability to switch off may mean that they run the risk of working themselves into the ground. The remedy encourages you to be more flexible mentally, and also to take a calming step back to relax.

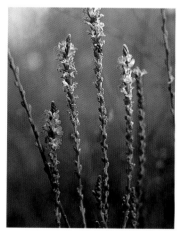

Harvesting
Vervain blooms in mid to late summer. It is best harvested young.

Datafile

BOTANICAL NAME
Verbena officinalis.

HABITAT
Dry, sunny pastures, wasteland, and roadsides.

PLANT DESCRIPTION
Vervain produces small, pale mauve or lilac flowers, which blossom from midsummer to early fall. The buds lower down on the plant open before the upper ones.

REMEDY PREPARATION
Sun method. Do not collect fading or dead flowers.

INDICATIONS FOR USE
Excessive zeal and commitment; obsession with one's own point of view to the exclusion of all others; sense of injustice leading to fanaticism; excessive energy; overdoing things; building up nervous tensions without a release for them.

WHAT TREATMENT SHOULD ACHIEVE
Vervain increases flexibility of mind, so that you can take account of other people's views, rather than always simply arguing your own. It will help you set limits to your efforts and allow yourself time to relax and rest.

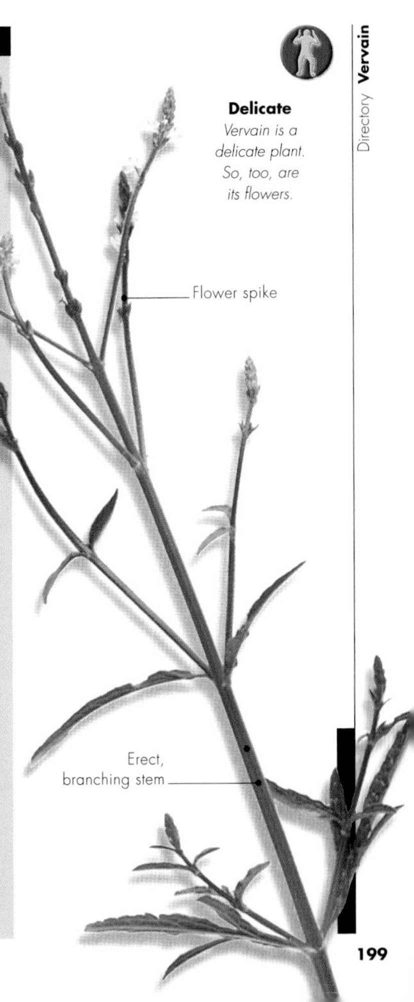

Delicate
Vervain is a delicate plant. So, too, are its flowers.

Flower spike

Erect, branching stem

199

The Vervain Remedy

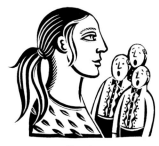

Listening
Vervain helps you to start listening to the views of others.

If you are a Vervain person, you are a perfectionist, and you also have a keen sense of natural justice. You are full of energy, too, which you are willing to throw into anything that you believe in, at the same time exerting all your powers to win others round to your point of view.

Although such enthusiasm can be infectious, there is a possibility that, if carried to extremes, it may be counterproductive. Instead of trying to get your way by persuasion—and accepting the occasional failure with good grace—you run the risk of becoming dogmatic, set in your ways, and unable to take on board anything that goes against your own particular viewpoint.

Getting things done the way you want may be becoming an end in itself, and you may find yourself growing more and more obsessive about it. If this happens, especially if you are not getting your own way, your stress levels may well rise to danger point as you push yourself ever harder. You may become a workaholic or a fanatic, unable to rest or to listen properly to other points of view.

Wasting energy

If you find yourself in this state, one thing should be clear to you: matters cannot be allowed to go on like this for ever. What you are running the risk of is exhausting all your reserves of energy, and your health may suffer as a result.

What is happening is that, rather than employing your energies productively, you may be squandering them in wasted effort. In your absolute determination to persuade others that you are right, for instance, you may well be letting things get out of control.

Taking time to pause

You are no longer open to argument, or to listen to and take account of any views that are contrary to your own. The more this goes on, the more likely it is that you will become increasingly stressed: when things do not work out, the result may well be a deep burning anger, which shows itself in renewed attempts to persuade people to see things your way.

The remedy will free you from the treadmill you have made for yourself, allowing you to rest and take time out so that your positive qualities can blossom.

The Negative State

The negative **Vervain** state is characterized by nervous tension, caused by excessive zeal and energy, resulting in overdoing things.

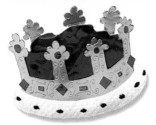

Natural leaders
Though Vine people are natural leaders, the risk is that they may try to impose their will on others.

VINE
Highly capable and strong, with tremendous willpower and presence of mind, Vine people are natural leaders. If, however, you fall into a negative Vine state, the danger is that the pluses all become minuses. From merely thinking that you know what is best for others, you may end up trying to pressure them to do what you think is best for them by sheer force of personality alone. The remedy brings Vine's positive aspects to the fore, so that, rather than dictate and impose, you recognize the value of winning over hearts and minds.

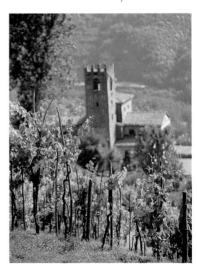

Remedy
Remedy makers avoid the use of cultivated vines when making the Vine remedy.

Datafile

BOTANICAL NAME
Vitis vinifera.

HABITAT
Mediterranean.

PLANT DESCRIPTION
Vine is a climber, which, when mature, grows to a height of 50 feet (15 meters) or more. Its flowers, which are small, green, and fragrant, grow in dense clusters. The flowering season varies with the climate, depending on where the vine is being grown.

REMEDY PREPARATION
Sun method.

INDICATIONS FOR USE
Being domineering and inflexible; trying to tyrannize others; riding roughshod over others and ignoring their opinions; forcing others to comply with your demands.

WHAT TREATMENT SHOULD ACHIEVE
The remedy helps to bring out positive Vine qualities to take the place of the negative ones. This means that you can take full advantage of your natural wisdom and the respect in which you are held to inspire and lead through example and persuasion, not by force.

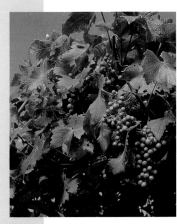

Tendrils
The grape vine climbs by means of tendrils.

The Vine Remedy

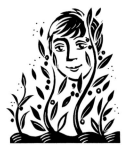

A positive force
*Vine will help you
exercise your powers of
leadership humanely.*

In the positive state, Vine people possess all the qualities that make good leaders, particularly in emergencies. They can be extremely useful people to know.

In the negative state, though, there is the risk that they will lose all sense of proportion, believing themselves to be totally infallible, sure that whatever it is they decide on, it has to be the right way to go. Rather than trying to persuade others of the virtues of their case, they will simply ride roughshod over them. Herein lies dictatorship—it is probable that both Adolf Hitler and Joseph Stalin, for instance, were in the negative Vine state.

People in this state never suffer from uncertainty, or doubt. If anything, they believe that they are doing others a favor by driving things through. They do not see that in reality they are being tyrannical or even cruel.

Dominating others

People in the negative Vine state have lost all sympathy for others. Instead, they rely on sheer willpower and drive to see them through to success as they take it upon themselves to tackle life and all its problems. Whatever the situation, they totally lack the ability to compromise. They cannot brook opposition or dissent. Everybody is forced to dance to their tune.

Provided that others see and do things their way, Vine people can get along with them. If this is not the case, however, they may resort to bullying (this particularly applies to their direct subordinates). It is particularly likely that they will be unable to resist the temptation to dictate to people with gentler, more submissive characters than their own—Centaury people, for instance, are often natural Vine victims. Vine people are past masters at laying down the law to others.

Transforming the picture

Taking the remedy, however, can spark off a radical transformation, as you start to realize that there is everything to be said for using your powers of leadership more wisely, humanely, and positively. You will no longer feel the need to be imperious and dictatorial. There will be no diminution of your natural authority—in fact, it is likely to be enhanced now it is being tempered by a new-found respect for the wishes and the rights of others.

The Negative State

The negative **Vine** state is characterized by a lack of sympathy or consideration for others and loss of a sense of proportion.

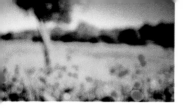

Beauty
The Beech remedy will help you
by injecting more beauty into life.

BEECH

According to Dr. Bach, Beech is the remedy for people who "feel the need to see more good and beauty in all that surrounds them." The sign of a negative Beech state is to lack tolerance of others, particularly of the ways in which they lead their lives. People like this are constant carpers and critics, quick to condemn rather than make any effort to understand. The remedy helps to generate tolerance. It also helps to deal with the irritable outbursts that may feature as part of a negative Beech state.

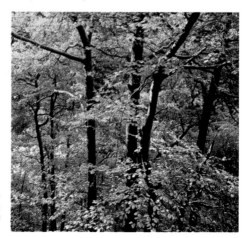

Height
Beech trees can reach
heights of 100 feet
(30 meters) when mature.

Datafile

BOTANICAL NAME
Fagus sylvatica.

HABITAT
Woodland.

PLANT DESCRIPTION
Beech flowers in mid- to late spring, at the same time as its leaves emerge. Male and female flowers grow on the same tree. The males, which are purplish brown, form hanging clusters on long stalks. Each female cluster consists of two flowers enclosed in a cup of overlapping scales.

REMEDY PREPARATION
Boiling method. Use young shoots, with newly opened leaves, as well as both male and female flowers.

INDICATIONS FOR USE
Sitting in judgment over others; being intolerant of other people's views and wishes; being constantly critical of others and everything they try to do.

WHAT TREATMENT SHOULD ACHIEVE
The remedy encourages you to see the good in others. It gives you the ability to be more tolerant and understanding. Now, you will be prepared to listen to others, paying attention to what they say. You will be able to work with them constructively, rather than spend your time constantly criticizing them for their supposed faults and shortcomings.

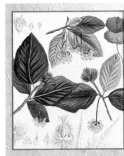

Fagus Sylvatica.

Harvesting
Beech should be harvested as soon as the flowers have opened fully.

The Beech Remedy

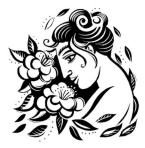

Tolerance

Beech promotes greater understanding and tolerance of others' views.

If you are a Beech person, you possess a well-developed sense of right and wrong and extremely high ethical and moral standards. Unfortunately, if you fall into a negative Beech state, you become so convinced of your own rectitude that, instead of respecting the right of others to have views and opinions, you become completely intolerant of them.

Consequently, your instant response is to criticize: you are simply not prepared to take the time to consider any opinions other than your own. Not only are you absolutely positive that what you want is best, but also that it is illogical for anyone else to argue against it. If this happens, you can be extremely destructive and condemnatory.

Running people down

What this means is that, in the eyes of other people, you are a constant, carping critic who is best avoided. Rather than trying to look at things positively, you tend to take a negative, judgemental view. As a result, you can come across to others as being arrogant, narrow-minded, and lacking in common humility and humanity.

Such reactions are not totally unjustified. As far as you are concerned, you are constantly on the lookout for other people's shortcomings. When you feel that you have discovered some, you are only too willing to criticize and condemn, rather than trying to be even slightly constructive. You seem to be incapable of putting yourself into other people's shoes and trying to appreciate their point of view. Although, on the surface, you may appear calm and patient, inwardly you may be seething with irritation, which even the minor idiosyncrasies of others can easily bring to the surface. You may be lonely as well, your harsh, intolerant attitudes cutting you off from companionship.

Gaining in tolerance

The remedy helps you to be, as Dr. Bach described it, "more tolerant, lenient, and understanding of the different way each individual and all things are working to their final perfection." You will come to appreciate that, in fact, there is a lot to be said for encouraging diversity. In addition, you will learn that you can only benefit by showing a willingness to learn from and help others.

The Negative State

The negative **Beech** state is characterized by intolerance of the wishes, opinions, and actions of others.

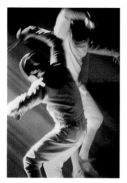

Perfectionism
Punishing yourself for failing to live up to your own standard is a typical negative Rock Water characteristic.

ROCK WATER
Rock Water is the odd one out among the Bach remedies, since it is the only one that is not derived from a plant. Instead, it consists of fresh, unpolluted water from healing springs or wells. You may need the remedy if, as part of a somewhat puritanical approach to life, you are taking things to extremes, punishing yourself if you are failing to live up to the standards that you have set for yourself, which may be unnaturally high. Rock Water eases the pressure by making you less rigid and more flexible without compromising your ideals and the efforts you are making to live up to them.

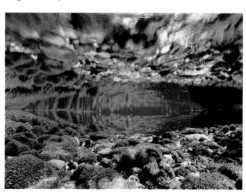

Wales
The water currently used by the Bach Centre to make Rock Water remedy comes from a source in Wales.

Datafile

SOURCE
Unpolluted, natural springs or wells.

REMEDY PREPARATION
Sun method.

INDICATIONS FOR USE
Playing the martyr; denying yourself even the simplest pleasures in life; punishing yourself if you stray from your predetermined path.

WHAT TREATMENT SHOULD ACHIEVE
The remedy encourages flexibility of thought. It gives you the ability to enjoy life and its experiences in a relaxed, calm way, while still upholding all your original high ideals.

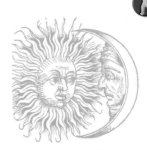

Sun method
The sun method is used when the sun is at the height of its power.

Preparation
To make the remedy, pure springwater is energized by the sun method.

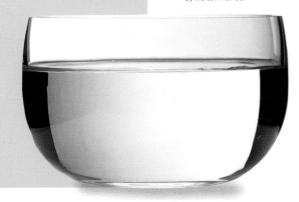

The Rock Water Remedy

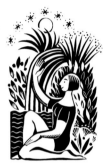

Flexibility
*Rock Water helps
you to temper high moral
standards with humanity.*

Rock Water will help you if you find yourself in danger of becoming a martyr to your beliefs. This is largely because you have allowed yourself to develop a rigid, inflexible personality that finds it impossible to compromise, even though, to others, it would seem natural common sense to at least consider doing so.

You will also be particularly hard on yourself. Just as nothing and no one can deflect you from the high ideals you have set for yourself, you will force yourself to try to live up to them at all costs. If necessary, as part of this quest for perfection, you will starve yourself of leisure and pleasure: like the Puritan fanatics of old, you will govern yourself with a rod of iron.

The quest itself can take many forms. For instance, it may well be one of your goals to be constantly in top mental and physical shape. You may have set your heart on becoming a star member of Mensa, or on entering and winning a prestigious marathon. Although you are not trying to influence others deliberately, you would like to be an example for them to emulate.

What you are missing

In this state, you may fail to realize that the self-coercion you are applying is leading you to suppress other important human needs. The mistake is to think that all the demands you are making on yourself, which may well become more and more exaggerated as time goes by, are the keys to self-enlightenment and eventual self-perfection. They are not necessarily the only way forward. Indeed, the pressure that they may end up putting you under could lead to stress, unhappiness, and self-reproach.

Reassessing your life

The Rock Water remedy will help you to reassess the situation. You will come to the realization that no one is perfect as the remedy helps you start a re-evaluation of the way you are living your life. This does not mean abandoning existing standards: rather, it means being prepared to keep an open, not a closed, mind. This way, you will be able to put preconceptions aside, so that, for example, you can make the most of new contacts and fresh new experiences, rather than refusing to accept that they have something useful to teach.

The Negative State

The negative **Rock Water** state is characterized by a quest for perfection and punishing yourself if you fail to achieve it.

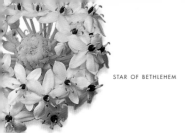

STAR OF BETHLEHEM

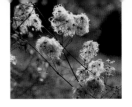

CLEMATIS

RESCUE REMEDY

The emergency mixture sold under the trade name Rescue Remedy is unquestionably the most widely known of all the 38 Bach flower remedies. It is a composite of five individual remedies that Dr. Bach himself devised—and carried with him—to be used specifically to help in emergencies and crises, when there simply would not be time to select specific remedies to meet the situation's needs.

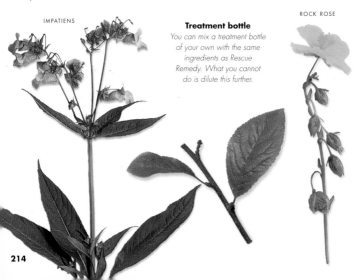

IMPATIENS

ROCK ROSE

Treatment bottle
You can mix a treatment bottle of your own with the same ingredients as Rescue Remedy. What you cannot do is dilute this further.

Datafile

RESCUE REMEDY CONSISTS OF
- Star of Bethlehem (for shock)
- Rock Rose (for terror and panic)
- Clematis (for faintness and unconsciousness)
- Impatiens (for mental stress, tension, and agitation)
- Cherry Plum (for desperation and loss of self-control)

Cream
You can add Rescue Remedy and Crab Apple to a lotion.

Rescue Remedy and water

Dosing
Sip a glass of diluted Rescue Remedy until the crisis is passed.

Rescue Remedy

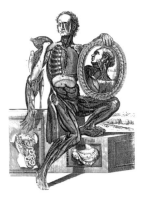

Emergency
*Rescue Remedy helps in
any emergency situation.*

Rescue Remedy will come to your
aid in any emergency, great or
small. Thousands of people across
the world who have turned to it in times
of crisis over the years can testify to its
effectiveness. Indeed, some people rely
on it exclusively practically all the time,
although, in fact, this is a mistake
(though not a serious one). This is not
because it is dangerous to take Rescue
Remedy longterm. It is not. Rather, if you

use it all the time, this indicates that you
need to use individually selected
remedies to deal with the causes of your
constant crises.

How Rescue Remedy evolved
In its original form, Rescue Remedy
consisted of Rock Rose, Clematis, and
Impatiens: Dr. Bach added the other
two remedies, Star of Bethlehem and
Cherry Plum, after their later discovery.
He used Rescue Remedy in 1933
to save the life of a drowning seaman,
who had been swept overboard during
a storm off the coast of Norfolk,
England, and it has been a firm standby ever since. Although Rescue Remedy
is a potent first-aid measure for use in
any emergency, it cannot supplant
skilled medical treatment, nor was
it designed to do so.

There are various ways of taking
Rescue Remedy, but the standard one is
to mix four drops of stock concentrate in
a glass of water and get the patient to
sip this frequently until calm. Alternatively,
if the patient is unable to do this, or is

unconscious, you can rub the energized water onto the lips, the gums, behind the ears, and on the wrists. If there is nothing available with which to dilute it, then you should apply Rescue Remedy neat to the lips, tongue, or gums.

You can also apply Rescue Remedy in diluted form directly to minor injuries, using it to bathe a painful area, or in compresses, applied hot or cold. In this case, use four drops to ½ quart (500 milliliters) of water.

Alternatively, you can use Rescue Cream, which is a homeopathically prepared cream containing Rescue Remedy and purifying Crab Apple. It was devised by Nora Weeks, Dr. Bach's original assistant, to make it easier to apply Rescue Remedy to the skin. It can be used to treat cuts and bruises and for skin problems of various kinds.

The Negative State

The negative state requiring **Rescue Remedy** is a crisis or emergency that needs immediate attention.

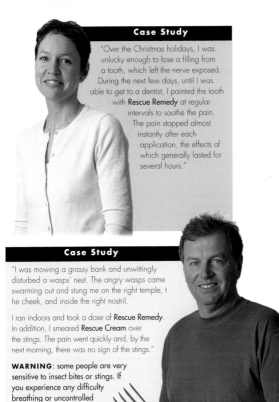

Case Study

"Over the Christmas holidays, I was unlucky enough to lose a filling from a tooth, which left the nerve exposed. During the next few days, until I was able to get to a dentist, I painted the tooth with **Rescue Remedy** at regular intervals to soothe the pain. The pain stopped almost instantly after each application, the effects of which generally lasted for several hours."

Case Study

"I was mowing a grassy bank and unwittingly disturbed a wasps' nest. The angry wasps came swarming out and stung me on the right temple, the cheek, and inside the right nostril.

I ran indoors and took a dose of **Rescue Remedy**. In addition, I smeared **Rescue Cream** over the stings. The pain went quickly and, by the next morning, there was no sign of the stings."

WARNING: some people are very sensitive to insect bites or stings. If you experience any difficulty breathing or uncontrolled swelling, or if you have a known sensitivity to insect stings, seek immediate medical attention.

FURTHER READING

BACH, DR. EDWARD, *The Twelve Healers and Other Remedies*, The C.W. Daniel Company Ltd.

BACH, DR. EDWARD, *Heal Thyself*, The C.W. Daniel Company Ltd.

BALL, STEFAN, *Principles of Bach Flower Remedies*, Thorsons.

BALL, STEFAN, *The Bach Remedies Workbook*, The C.W. Daniel Company Ltd.

BALL, STEFAN, *Bach Flower Remedies for Men*, The C.W. Daniel Company Ltd.

CHANCELLOR, PHILIP M., *Illustrated Handbook of the Bach Flower Remedies*, The C.W. Daniel Company Ltd.

EVANS, JANE, *Introduction to the Benefits of the Bach Flower Remedies*, The C.W. Daniel Company Ltd.

HOWARD, JUDY, *The Bach Flower Remedies Step by Step*, The C.W. Daniel Company Ltd.

HOWARD, JUDY, *Bach Flower Remedies for Women*, The C.W. Daniel Company Ltd.

HOWARD, JUDY, *Growing Up with Bach Flower Remedies*, The C.W. Daniel Company Ltd.

HOWARD, JUDY, *The Story of Mount Vernon*, The Dr. Edward Bach Centre.

HYNE-JONES, T.W., *Dictionary of the Bach Flower Remedies*, The C.W. Daniel Company Ltd.

RAMSELL, JOHN, *Questions and Answers*, The C.W. Daniel Company Ltd.

RAMSELL, JOHN AND HOWARD, JUDY, eds., *The Original Writings of Edward Bach*, The C.W. Daniel Company Ltd.

WEEKS, NORA AND BULLEN, VICTOR, *The Bach Flower Remedies*, The C.W. Daniel Company Ltd.

WHEELER, F.J., *The Bach Remedies Repertory*, The C.W. Daniel Company Ltd.

The Dr. Edward Bach Centre publishes a Newsletter three times a year. It also distributes an audio cassette, *Getting to Know the Bach Flower Remedies*, and two videos: *The Light that Never Goes Out: The Story of the Bach Flower Remedies* and *Bach Flower Remedies: A Further Understanding*. It also publishes a set of pictorial reference cards, illustrated in color with descriptions and information about each remedy.

USEFUL ADDRESSES

For further information about the remedies; details of educational programs and other activities; lists of registered Bach practitioners worldwide; and general health advice, you should contact the Dr. Edward Bach Centre, Mount Vernon, Bakers Lane, Sotwell, Oxfordshire OX10 0PZ, UK. The Centre can give free advice over the telephone (00 44 1491 834678) or you can contact them in writing or e-mail (bach@bachcentre.com). There is also a regularly updated website, which features information about the remedies, practitioner details, background on Dr. Bach and his work, frequently asked questions and answers, and more. The URL is http://www.bachcentre.com. To find out more about training in the US and around the world, contact the Dr. Edward Bach Foundation (Bach International Educational Program) at Mount Vernon (the e-mail address is foundation@bachcentre.com).

The worldwide distributor for the Bach Flower Remedies is:
A Nelson & Co.,
Broadheath House,
83 Parkside
London SW19 5LP, UK
(tel: 00 44 (0)20 8780 4200)

In the US, for more information on flower essences contact:
The Flower Essence Society,
PO Box 459, Nevada City, CA 95959
(tel: 800 736 9222)

In Canada, there are two national distributors:
Alypsis, PO Box 2465, Peterborough, Ontario K9J 7Y8 (tel: 00 1 705 749 1894)
Christmas Natural Foods, 201-8173 128th Street, Surrey, British Columbia V3W 4G1 (tel: 00 1 604 581 8881)

For details of the Bach International Education Program, contact:
The Balnea Institute,
383 6th Concession East,
PO Box 82061, Waterdown,
Ontario L0R 2M0
(tel: 00 1 905 689 3329)

In the US, the national distributor is:
Nelson Bach USA,
100 Research Drive,
Wilmington, MA 01887
(tel: 00 1 978 988 3833)
Their website URL is http://www.nelsonbach.com which also links to details of Bach Educational Program courses in the US.

INDEX

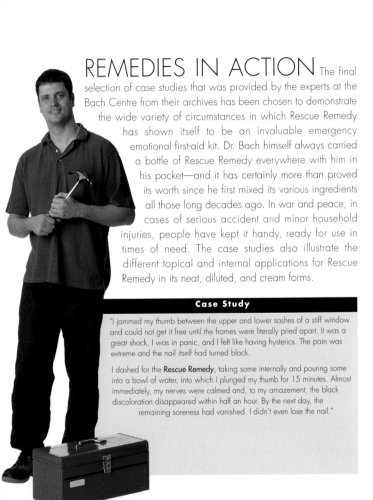

REMEDIES IN ACTION

The final selection of case studies that was provided by the experts at the Bach Centre from their archives has been chosen to demonstrate the wide variety of circumstances in which Rescue Remedy has shown itself to be an invaluable emergency emotional first-aid kit. Dr. Bach himself always carried a bottle of Rescue Remedy everywhere with him in his pocket—and it has certainly more than proved its worth since he first mixed its various ingredients all those long decades ago. In war and peace, in cases of serious accident and minor household injuries, people have kept it handy, ready for use in times of need. The case studies also illustrate the different topical and internal applications for Rescue Remedy in its neat, diluted, and cream forms.

Case Study

"I jammed my thumb between the upper and lower sashes of a stiff window and could not get it free until the frames were literally pried apart. It was a great shock, I was in panic, and I felt like having hysterics. The pain was extreme and the nail itself had turned black.

I dashed for the **Rescue Remedy**, taking some internally and pouring some into a bowl of water, into which I plunged my thumb for 15 minutes. Almost immediately, my nerves were calmed and, to my amazement, the black discoloration disappeared within half an hour. By the next day, the remaining soreness had vanished. I didn't even lose the nail."